QUESTIONS OF SEX

Here is a comprehensive selection of the questions about sex most often found in the postbags and files of doctors, counsellors, clinics and advice columns.

There are general questions about sexuality and puberty; questions about techniques, birth control and sexually transmitted diseases; as well as sections on gay sex and the legal aspects of sex.

Presented in a straightforward, sympathetic and factual way, the answers will allow people to feel confident enough to explore their own sexuality and decide what is right for them.

Also by The Diagram Group, and available from NEL:

SEX: A USER'S MANUAL

The Diagram Group

Consultants	Dr Sol Gordon Carol G Wells Beryl Heather
Editors	Sue Bosanko Joanna Evans
Editorial assistant	Annabel Else
Indexer	David Harding
Art director	Richard Hummerstone
Art staff	Joe Bonello, Richard Czapnik, Brian Hewson, Johanna Lidman, Jerry Watkiss, Marlene Williamson, Galina Zolfaghari

The authors and editors of the Diagram Group wish to acknowledge their debt to the many individuals and institutions whose detailed research projects into sexual topics have provided data for this book.

Questions of Sex

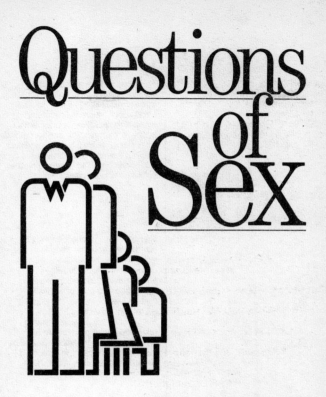

THE DIAGRAM GROUP

NEW ENGLISH LIBRARY
Hodder and Stoughton

Copyright © 1988
Diagram Visual Information Ltd
195 Kentish Town Road
London NW5 8SY

First published in Great Britain in 1989
by NEL paperbacks

This book is sold subject to the condition that it shall not, by way of trade or otherwise, be lent, re-sold, hired out or otherwise circulated without the publisher's prior consent in any form of binding or cover other than that in which it is published and without a similar condition including this condition being imposed on the subsequent purchaser.

No part of this publication may be reproduced or transmitted in any form or by any means, electronically or mechanically, including photocopying, recording or any information storage or retrieval system, without either the prior permission in writing from the publisher or a licence, permitting restricted copying. In the United Kingdom such licences are issued by the Copyright Licensing Agency, 33–34 Alfred Place, London WC1E 7DP.

British Library C.I.P.

Questions of sex.
 1. Sex relations
 I. Diagram Group
 306.7

ISBN 0 450 43078 2

Typeset by Bournetype, Bournemouth, England.
Printed and bound in Great Britain for Hodder and Stoughton paperbacks, a division of Hodder and Stoughton Ltd., Mill Road, Dunton Green, Sevenoaks, Kent TN13 2YA (Editorial Office: 47 Bedford Square, London WC1B 3DP) by Cox & Wyman Ltd., Reading.

Foreword

Sexual activity is a natural aspect of life, and is as important and necessary as eating, breathing, thinking or dreaming. Our bodies were assembled from neither unsavoury, unmentionable nor unrelated parts, but they are the result of an evolutionary process which has produced a design capable of performing specific functions.

Most boys and girls feel a sense of uncertainty or inadequacy at some stage in their adolescence, and often attribute the cause of their problems to lack of experience. However, many adults also have similar problems which do not necessarily disappear with age. Rewarding sexual experience stems from an inner understanding and sympathy between your partner and yourself. Life can often be unhappy for the adolescent since ignorance often breeds fear. Understanding the functions of the body and the mind enables you to feel more confident of both your physical and mental reactions. There are two ways to learn – the first is from your own experiences, the second by considering the experiences of other people. Both failure and success contribute to these experiences. Misinformation can sometimes be more harmful than no information at all since we may either act upon incorrect assumptions, or follow advice mistakenly given by others. On the other hand, having nobody to talk to can produce a fear that what we are experiencing is in some way abnormal or harmful. The solution resides in the ability to know which questions to ask in order to receive the answers required.

In most forms of sexual activity what matters most is making both yourself and your partner feel happy, safe in the knowledge that your activities are not harmful to each other. Socially acceptable activities, as condoned by friends, parents or society in general, do not always provide the framework for your sexual experience. A relationship with a partner who is much older or younger, or of a different race, or of the same sex, may be the right course to follow. Throughout history no society has ever fully answered the questions relating to sex, but has tried to pass on the knowledge gained by adults in the hope that the children can avoid unnecessary doubts and fears.

When opportunities for sexual experience occur, think carefully of the spiritual and psychological consequences of your actions and not simply the physical results. Sexual activity should never be an exploitation of your partner, rather a considered response to their needs.

All the questions in QUESTIONS OF SEX have been collected from the files and postbags of doctors, counsellors, clinics and advice columnists. They are all real questions about growing up, emotional and physical development, the facts of life and sexuality – questions that can cause anxiety if left unanswered. Above all, they are questions which people often find difficult to ask, let alone answer.

Whatever the question, QUESTIONS OF SEX answers it in a straightforward and factual way. The facts are presented so that the readers have enough background knowledge to make up their own mind on what they should do. In answering the questions, our concern is to inform and reassure, to point out responsibilities and likely consequences, but not to make judgments on behaviour.

QUESTIONS OF SEX is divided into seven sections: **Section one:** AM I NORMAL? includes general questions on sex and human sexuality; **Section two:** GROWING UP includes general questions on puberty and separate questions on growing up for girls and boys; **Section three:** THE ART OF LOVING includes questions on techniques, tastes and sexual difficulties; **Section four:** THE QUESTION OF PREGNANCY includes questions on the likelihood of pregnancy, methods of birth control, sterilization and abortion; **Section five:** is about GAY RELATIONSHIPS; **Section six:** concerns SEXUALLY TRANSMITTED DISEASES and **Section seven** focuses on SEX AND THE LAW. There is also a glossary of words which might present problems, an index, and a list of addresses of clinics, organizations and health centres.

Useful addresses

Pregnancy, birth control and sexual problems

Brook Advisory Centre
153A East Street (Head Office)
London SE17 2SD
Tel: 01 708 1234

Branches: Avon, Birmingham,
Burnley, Coventry, Edinburgh,
Liverpool, London

The Family Planning Association (FPA)
27–35 Mortimer Street (Head Office)
London W1
Tel: 01 636 7866

Help and advice on AIDS

Terence Higgins Trust
BM/AIDS
London WC1N 3XX
Tel: 01 242 1010 help line
VISTEL (for the deaf and
hard of hearing) 01 405 2463
3–10pm daily

Health advice (free leaflets, etc)

Health Education Council
78 New Oxford Street
London WC1A 1AH
Tel: 01 631 0930

Health Information Trust
(Started by College of Health)
Tel: 01 980 4848

Help and advice on rape

Rape Crisis Centre
PO Box 69
London WC1
Tel: 01 278 3956 (office hours)
01 837 1600 (24 hours)

Help and advice on gay relationships

Gay Switchboard
BM Switchboard
London WC1N 3XX
Tel: 01 837 7324

Special Clinics (see also telephone directories under Venereal diseases)

James Pringle House
73/5 Charlotte Street
London W1
Tel: 01 380 9141

Marlborough Clinic
Royal Free Hospital
Pond Street
London NW3
Tel: 01 794 0500

Praed Street Clinic
St Mary's Hospital
Praed Street
London W2
Tel: 01 725 1697

University College Hospital
Gower Street
London WC1
Tel: 01 387 9300

Contents

Pages 10–33

Section one:
AM I NORMAL?

Pages 34–77

Section two:
GROWING UP

Pages 78–105

Section three:
THE ART OF LOVING

Pages 106–143

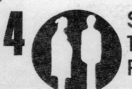

Section four:
THE QUESTION OF PREGNANCY

Pages 144–153

5  **Section five:**
GAY RELATIONSHIPS

Pages 154–173

6 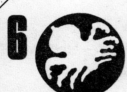 **Section six:**
SEXUALLY TRANSMITTED DISEASES

Pages 174–185

7 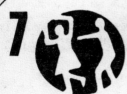 **Section seven:**
SEX AND THE LAW

Pages 186–188 **GLOSSARY**

Pages 189–192 **INDEX**

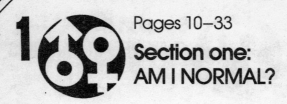

Section one: AM I NORMAL?

Pages 10–33

- Why do people have sex? **12**
- Are people from other countries different when it comes to having sex? **13**
- If sex is something beautiful, why do people snigger or get embarrassed? **14**
- Why do doctors and teachers use different words about sex from those my friends and I use? **14**
- Why do we get sex education in biology classes? **15**
- How old do you have to be before you can have sex? **16**
- How old do you have to be before you can buy condoms? **17**
- Do boys need sex more than girls? **17**
- Why do boys enjoy looking at pictures of naked women? **18**
- Are girls just pretending not to be turned on by pictures of naked men? **18**
- When girls say no, do they really mean yes? **19**
- Are girls who carry contraceptives promiscuous? **19**
- What's so bad about promiscuity? **20**
- What is frigidity? **20**
- My boyfriend wants to have sex but I don't. Am I frigid? **21**
- How soon should you let your boyfriend go all the way? **22**
- Is it okay for a girl to make a pass at a boy? **23**
- If I feel sexy about more than one boy at a time, does it mean I'm a nymphomaniac? **23**
- My boyfriend likes French kissing but I don't. Is there something wrong with me? **24**
- My friends all talk about the number of times they've done it, but I've never had sex. Am I normal? **24**

- I'm not very interested in sex. Am I normal? **25**
- If you want to have sex with someone, are you in love? **25**
- Do you always want to have sex with someone you're in love with? **26**
- Are some people better at sex than others? **26**
- Why do my parents get embarrassed when I ask them about sex? **27**
- My father doesn't seem to mind the idea of my brother having sex, but he makes a fuss about me because I'm a girl. Why is this? **28**
- Why do they tell sportsmen not to masturbate or have sex before a game? **29**
- Why is my mother against my having an older boyfriend? **29**
- I am disabled and my parents think I shouldn't know about sex. What should I do? **30**
- I think my parents are still having sex. Shouldn't they have stopped by now? **30**
- My grandad wants to get married again. Why are my parents so shocked? **31**
- What types of sex are wrong? **31**
- Why do people have sex with prostitutes? **32**
- What is meant by the term 'sexual perversion'? **33**

Section one: AM I NORMAL?

Why do people have sex?

Sex, at its most basic, is nature's way of ensuring the continuation of species. Animals don't think about it: they respond to changing levels of sex hormones which stimulate (or curb) the reproductive urge. But in human beings thi response is complicated by thoughts and feelings – all the higher mental processes which distinguish us from the rest of the animal world. Certainly we have sex to have babies, but as the only species capable of having sex at any time (animals only mate when the female comes on heat), we do it for all sorts of other reasons, too. We have sex because it is pleasurable, because we think it is expected of us, to prove ourselves or because we're too frightened to say no. It is only as we mature that we come to experience sex as the centre of a loving relationship, a true bond between two people.

Are people from other countries different when it comes to having sex?

The basic sex drive is a universal experience, but what turns people on differs from culture to culture. In societies where people wear few clothes, for example, the sight of a woman's breasts or a man's penis does not have the automatic sexual association that it would in Europe. In some parts of the world – Tonga, for instance – fat women are considered more desirable than thin ones. A position for having sex which is popular in one country may not be acceptable in another.

The rules and customs which govern sexual behaviour vary enormously. Relationships or activities may be either encouraged or disapproved of, depending on where you are. Psychiatrists and sociologists, biologists, religious leaders and politicians have all, at some time, defined acceptable sexual behaviour, each claiming his or her view to be the right one. What no one doubts is that sexuality is an essential part of being human.

Section one: AM I NORMAL?

If sex is something beautiful, why do people snigger or get embarrassed?

Sex still makes some people feel uncomfortable and embarrassed partly because it has been associated for so long with unacceptable and 'dirty' feelings. Sniggering is sometimes a way of covering up these feelings. Embarrassment also comes from the secrecy surrounding the sexual act. Secrets mean you have done something wrong. In societies where sex has been open and free from ideas of guilt, it is accepted much more easily as being normal and natural.

Why do doctors and teachers use different words about sex from those that my friends and I use?

Scientists are trained to use words which are precise in their meaning and, so far as possible, free from emotion. Doctors, for instance, describe entry into the vagina by the penis as coition. The word may not be attractive, but it means just what it says. The terms they use for the sex organs (as well as for other parts of the body) and for what we do with them have to be specific. Popular terms, on the other hand, are often vague: having it off, for instance, may mean different things to different people, depending on their sexual preferences.

Teachers may choose to refer to parts of the body and to sexual activities in scientific language partly because it is more precise. It also makes the subject more impersonal – less embarrassing and less likely to raise awkward questions.

Why do we get sex education in biology classes?

The main reason that sex education may be taught in biology classes is that, as an academic subject at least, it belongs there. Human reproduction is a normal biological process – one of the vital functions. Biology teachers can compare the reproductive mechanisms of plants and animals and of higher and lower species; they can describe fertility cycles and the mechanics of copulation. But, as everyone now agrees, there is more to sex education than the facts of life. Just as important is the emotional and social side, the need to find answers to those difficult questions about how we and others do (or should) behave. It is for this reason that some schools now give sex education its own place in the syllabus, so that the whole subject – facts and feelings, rights and reponsibilities – can be given the time it needs.

Section one: AM I NORMAL?

How old do you have to be before you can have sex?

Some people – men and women – may never reach the maturity needed to enjoy a good sexual relationship; others mature while they are still in their teens. It is for you to judge yourself and to decide if and when you are ready to have sex, bearing in mind that it is illegal for a boy to have sex with a girl under 16.

It would be handy to have a set of guidelines for sex (as it would for any other human activity) rather than having to use your own judgment. Today, boys and girls are increasingly having to make their own decisions about sex, and it's never easy. When it comes to deciding if, and when, to have sex, remember that losing your virginity is an important landmark in your life. In doing so, you will experience a new and powerful way of expressing your love and affection. Along with pleasure, however, come demands. A relationship needs honesty between the partners and a certain amount of openness: secrecy often only leads to feelings of guilt. You should not only respect your sex partner, you should be able to respect yourself too. In addition, you have to accept the consequences of a sexual relationship – the fact that you are developing a unique intimacy with another person and that sex without contraception could lead to pregnancy. In other words, maturity in this case means being able to look to the future rather than only considering your immediate pleasure.

How old do you have to be before you can buy condoms?

There is no age limit to buying condoms (sheaths) and shop assistants have no right to ask you how old you are when they sell them to you. In fact, if you are old enough (and sensible enough) to use contraceptives, sales staff won't think your purchase at all strange. Sheaths are also available from slot machines in some public lavatories, but this is not a good way to get hold of them: the rubber perishes after a while, and you have no way of knowing how long they've been stored.

Do boys need sex more than girls?

The sex drive is a basic urge of human beings, and neither sex can claim more of it than the other. Some experts believe that boys often experience the strongest sex urges in their late teens, while women's sexual feelings are strongest in their thirties and forties. Others disagree and take the view that people's sexual feelings vary so much that it is impossible to generalize about any particular group.

Section one: AM I NORMAL?

Why do boys enjoy looking at pictures of naked women?

Most boys and men can become sexually aroused when looking at pictures of naked women or watching sexy films and by having sexual fantasies. Adolescent boys usually have frequent erections, responding very quickly to stimuli like these. Arousal is a pleasurable feeling so boys enjoy looking at these pictures.

Are girls just pretending not to be turned on by pictures of naked men?

Boys may find it hard to believe that girls are rarely aroused by the sight of naked men, live or in print, but it's true. Girls are usually only turned on by boys to whom they are emotionally attracted. Even then, they respond best to direct sexual stimuli, to being caressed.

When girls say no, do they really mean yes?

If a girl says no, then it is safe to assume she means no. If you feel you have to coax, wheedle, tease, nag or even threaten your girlfriend into having sex, then you are only thinking of yourself. Girls have a right to be taken as seriously as boys. If you care at all about her, you'll respect her decision and not assume she is merely playing hard to get.

Are girls who carry contraceptives promiscuous?

No, merely having contraceptives is not a mark of promiscuity. A girl who carries (and uses) contraceptives is accepting responsibility for her actions and showing that she cares both for herself and for her boyfriend.

What's so bad about promiscuity?

Promiscuity – flitting from one sexual partner to the next in quick succession – is regrettable for several reasons. For a start, the risk of sexually transmitted disease is greatly increased. Then there are the emotional considerations – not least the fact that you can develop no sense of caring or commitment if you sleep around. The most promiscuity offers is instant sexual gratification, not the fulfilment which comes from a single, loving relationship. Promiscuous people are often very lonely indeed.

What is frigidity?

Frigidity is an unhelpful term, applied only to women, which simply means coldness – an indifference to sex amounting sometimes to an aversion. It is a term which is often wrongly used. For instance, it is wrong to describe a girl who doesn't seem very interested in sex as frigid. It is more likely that either she is not yet ready for sex or she simply doesn't fancy the person making the sexual approaches.

True frigidity is nearly always the result of some bad sexual or emotional experience. People who have suffered in this way may want to respond in a loving manner, but they have an emotional block over sex, which makes them freeze up. Frigidity can usually be overcome by sympathetic counselling and love and understanding from the partner.

My boyfriend wants to have sex but I don't. Am I frigid?

A girl may begin to have sex with her boyfriend before she really wants to because of psychological pressures on her. He may threaten to leave her or claim that she doesn't really love him. Or he may accuse her of being frigid. If you feel sexual desire but have made a decision not to have sex you are not frigid. You probably have a strong sense of what is right for you.

Section one: AM I NORMAL?

How soon should you let your boyfriend go all the way?

There used to be an easy answer to this question: on your wedding night. For many reasons, this is no longer satisfactory for many young people, who now prefer to make their own decisions. This puts other pressures on teenagers. Despite the general acceptance of premarital sex, certain old ways persist, and the boy is almost always the one who asks to have sex. Few girls agree to have sex with a casual date, so the question comes up after two people have been going steady for a while.

You may agree to have sex because every one else has (or have they?). Or because you are curious. Or because heavy petting becomes foreplay which may lead to intercourse. You should consider what taking this step means to your future and not just what you feel or want in the immediate situation. You are entitled to pay attention to your own long-term feelings, however, and if you feel uneasy, unsure or guilty, this may not be the right time. Satisfying sex is never something a boy does to a girl, but something you share with each other.

Is it okay for a girl to make a pass at a boy?

In theory there's no reason at all why a girl shouldn't let a boy know she fancies him. Some people, however, still frown on a girl taking the first step in starting a relationship. Their disapproval is rooted in the old belief that 'nice' girls don't do it – and certainly don't make sexual demands for themselves. But the fact is that girls have as much need of – and as much right to – a loving sexual relationship as boys. So why shouldn't they speak up?

If I feel sexy about more than one boy at a time, does it mean I'm a nymphomaniac?

No, it simply means you're young and healthy. One of the effects of hormone activity around puberty is to make the young person – boy or girl – feel very randy at times. It's admitted in boys, of course: no one thinks it's at all unusual for a boy to fancy more than one girl. But people are quick to label girls who admit to normal, healthy sexuality. Don't worry about them – or it. These intense feelings of yours will soon pass.

Section one: AM I NORMAL?

My boyfriend likes French kissing, but I don't. Is their something wrong with me?

Kissing as portrayed in the movies and on television may seem to be an expression of romantic love, but French kissing (or deep kissing as it's sometimes known) can be very sexy and intimate. If a girl doesn't really love the boy who's kissing her, French kissing can seem the opposite of exciting. By explaining that she is not ready for it, a girl can give the relationship time to develop so that she, as well as the boy, can enjoy kissing.

My friends all talk about the number of times they've done it, but I've never had sex. Am I normal?

You are not only normal but probably more honest than the rest, for the chances are some of this talk is just boasting. The reason boys in particular feel the need to talk in this way is all to do with growing up. In Western society we have no ceremony equivalent to the initiation rites of some cultures to mark the arrival of adulthood. The value of such ceremonies is in showing everyone that the child has become a man or woman. So, since having sex is one of the signs of adulthood, some people feel the need to boast to show the world they've grown up.

I'm not very interested in sex. Am I normal?

There is no set age or school year when you suddenly become interested in sex. The way you feel has a lot to do with the level of sex hormones – oestrogen in girls, testoterone in boys. As the ovaries or testes (the primary sex organs) produce more hormones, your awareness of your sexuality will gradually increase; and then you will also become aware of the sexuality of others. If you are very involved in schoolwork, or spend a lot of time practising a musical instrument or playing a competitive sport, you may be developing dramatically in other directions at the moment. As time goes on, however, your sexuality will almost certainly become more apparent to you. If, however, you find the whole subject a great worry, you should try and talk about it to some responsible adults.

If you want to have sex with someone, are you in love?

You do not have to be in love to be turned on by someone. Many people are drawn to each other sexually, even though they know they could never really love each other. When, after puberty, you begin to develop your own sexuality, you may find yourself attracted to other people – classmates, pop stars, teachers, friends, even complete strangers. This intensity of feeling may be overwhelming, especially when it first happens. It takes time and experience to adjust to these new emotions, but gradually you should find yourself able to deal with them.

Section one: AM I NORMAL?

Do you always want to have sex with someone you're in love with?

Theoretically, you could have a platonic relationship – with no physical side at all – with the person you love. However, people in love often want to hold and touch one another, and sex is an extension of this feeling. They want to give themselves totally to their partner and not hold back in any way.

Are some people better at sex than others?

Sex isn't something to be judged like an athletic performance. To be good at sex, you need first of all to be sensitive to your partner's needs and feelings. Experience helps of course, but no amount of practice or experimentation can override the need to know and care about the other person. Even inexperienced partners can be 'good at sex' if they love each other enough to work at finding ways of giving pleasure and satisfaction.

Why do my parents get embarrassed when I ask them about sex?

You must remember that attitudes to sex have changed in recent years. After all, not long ago sex was never mentioned in public. People were too embarrassed to talk about it – it wasn't nice.

Today, even people who do not hold these outdated views may still find it difficult to answer questions about sex. For sexual relationships are very personal and go far beyond the physical; they have an important emotional element too, and it is never easy to talk about personal things and the way you feel. Families who are not used to talking about how they feel may find it very hard to discuss sex.

Section one: AM I NORMAL?

My father doesn't seem to mind the idea of my brother having sex, but he makes a fuss about me because I'm a girl. Why is this?

You may well be puzzled by the difference in your father's attitudes towards you and your brother. But you must remember that there are still double standards at work in our society: that boys are expected to be sexually adventurous from an early age, while girls are supposed to remain pure at least until they are grown up, if not until they are married. Bear in mind, too, that fathers tend to put their daughters on a pedestal and to be reluctant to see them become a woman and run the risk of becoming pregnant. Their inclination is to be overprotective towards daughters, while sons are free to have sexual adventures. It's a common reaction perhaps, but hard to live with if you're a girl.

Why do they tell sportsmen not to masturbate or have sex before a game?

It is probably a throwback to the old idea that sex (and masturbation in particular) is weakening, draining you of some vital force. This, of course, is rubbish: masturbating or having sex once requires no more energy than going up a flight of stairs. But obviously a team manager wouldn't want his players making love all night so they were too shattered next day to give their best on the sports field.

Why is my mother against my having an older boyfriend?

No doubt the last thing you want is advice from your mother (or any other adult) who seems to be out to spoil your fun. It is, after all, flattering to have the attentions of an older man who makes you feel grown up. But, while you see yourself as being mature, your mother thinks that you've got a long way to go yet. She probably feels uneasy about your going around with someone who may be one step ahead of you in every way and whom you are perhaps too immature to judge properly. He may be influencing you to do things (not just sex) or behave in a way which you are not yet ready for.

Section one: AM I NORMAL?

I am disabled and my parents think I shouldn't know about sex. What should I do?

Every adult has the right to have a satisfying sexual relationship. Learning about sex when you are young is an important step in this direction. Unfortunately, some people have the idea that there is something 'not nice' about sex for disabled people. This is really their problem not yours, for a disabled person has as much right to love and sex as anyone else. Tell your parents you have a right to know about sex or if you or they feel they can't help you, approach one of your teachers, your doctor, even a physiotherapist whom you trust, who can talk to you, give you helpful literature to read, or suggest someone else who can give you the information you need.

I think my parents are still having sex. Shouldn't they have stopped by now?

There is no age at which people automatically become 'past it'. One of the aspects of maturing is coming to recognize your parents as human beings with needs of all kinds, including sexual ones. It is normal for couples to have sex throughout their life together, and a good sexual relationship is usually inseparable from a good marriage.

My grandad wants to get married again. Why are my parents so shocked?

The relationship between a man and a woman is one of the most fulfilling parts of life at any age, whether at 18 or 80, and grandparents have as much right to love and sex as their children and grandchildren. Disapproval of this basic fact of life may be a sign that your parents haven't yet come to terms with aging.

What types of sex are wrong?

The matter of right or wrong types of sex is another question of attitudes to sex in general. There is no checklist of approved practices. Each person must decide for him or herself. The only hard and fast rule is that sex must always be voluntary and never do violence – physical or psychological – to yourself or your partner. If you are doing something that humiliates and hurts your partner it is wrong. If your partner forces you to do something you don't want to, this, too, is unacceptable. Physical violence leaves not only physical marks: it leaves emotional scars as well and these may never fade.

Section one: AM I NORMAL?

Why do people have sex with prostitutes?

There are many reasons why people have sex with prostitutes, who are mostly women but there are male prostitutes and homosexual prostitutes also. Often there is more to the casual meeting between prostitute and client than just physical pleasure. Some people go to prostitutes because they are lonely, or trapped in an unhappy marriage, or because they do not want emotional involvement in their sexual relationship. Prostitution may help these people, but buying sex for money cannot buy affection and caring as well, and there is also the danger of catching a sexually transmitted disease.

What is meant by the term 'sexual perversion'?

It is very difficult to know what people mean when they use this phrase. Strictly speaking, it means having a preference for a sexual practice which is not typical. But then, what is typical? For, as well-known research documents like the Kinsey Report have shown, many, many people go in for oddities of some kind. A prude may describe oral sex or even sex with the woman on top as perversion. In fact, some people's attitudes are so limited that they regard any sexual activity which is not intercourse in the 'missionary position' (preferably with the lights off) as perverted.

More reasonably, the phrase sexual perversion should be kept for sexual behaviour which is extreme and anti-social. In particular it is perverse to want to involve someone in sexual practices which cause them physical or psychological harm. Rape is a good example of this.

2

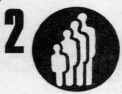

Pages 34–77

Section two: GROWING UP

- What is puberty? **36**
- When does puberty occur? **36**
- Are puberty and adolescence the same thing? **37**
- If sexual maturity starts with puberty, why did I get pubic hair when I was 10? **37**
- Why do my friends have hair on their bodies when I don't? **38**
- Why do boys' voices break but not girls'? **40**
- I haven't put on weight. Why don't my jeans fit any more? **40**
- When does the womb reach its full size? **42**
- When does a girl become fertile? **43**
- How does the egg get into the womb? **44**
- Why do girls have periods? **45**
- Why am I the only girl in my class who hasn't started periods? **46**
- My friend has her period every 28 days, but I never know when I'm going to start. Should I see a doctor? **46**
- What should I do to make my periods regular? **47**
- How can you tell when your period is going to start? **48**
- What is PMT? **49**
- Is it okay to do games when I have my period? **50**
- How can you use a tampon if you're still a virgin? **50**
- How do I know which size tampons to use? **51**
- I have trouble using tampons. How will I ever make love? **52**
- Can you 'lose' a tampon? **53**
- Will tampons make me ill? **53**
- My periods have stopped and I am growing facial hair. Is something wrong? **54**

- If I miss a period, am I pregnant? **54**
- Can all women have babies? **55**
- What is a clitoris and where is it? **56**
- Why do I get wet when I think about making love? **58**
- Can girls have wet dreams? **58**
- Vaginal deodorants make me itch. Do I need to use them? **59**
- One of my breasts seems to be growing larger than the other. What's wrong? **59**
- My breasts are too small. Can't I do something to make them grow? **60**
- Can you have a baby if you have small breasts? **60**
- If I don't wear a bra, will I be able to breastfeed when I have a baby? **61**
- What colour should my nipples be? **61**
- My nipples are flat. Is there something wrong with them? **62**
- When should you start checking your breasts for lumps? **62**
- Can men get breast cancer? **63**
- Can men's breasts produce milk? **63**
- My penis looks so small. Will I be able to have sex? **64**
- How can I make my penis bigger? **64**
- Are the testicles as important as the penis? **66**
- Why are my testicles different sizes? **66**
- My little brother is having an operation for an undescended testicle. What does this mean? **68**
- Where do sperms come from? **69**
- How much sperm should come out when you come? **70**
- Can you ever use up all the sperm the body can produce? **70**
- What happens to the sperm that aren't used up? **71**
- Do all men ejaculate? **71**
- Can you ejaculate without an erection? **72**
- How old do you have to be to have an erection? **74**
- It's very embarrassing to feel myself getting an erection when there are other people around. What can I do to stop it? **75**
- I don't remember having a sexy dream, so why were my pyjamas wet when I woke up? **75**
- Do wet dreams hurt? **76**
- I'm worried in case I have wet dream when I'm staying at my grandma's and she finds out. How can I stop having them? **76**
- Do semen and pee ever get mixed together since they both come out of the same place? **77**
- My breasts are getting bigger. Has something gone wrong? **77**

Section two: GROWING UP

What is puberty?

Puberty is the point in human development when the reproductive organs start working: girls ovulate for the first time and boys can ejaculate.

When does puberty occur?

The precise age of puberty differs from person to person. The average age for menstruation to begin for girls is between 11 and 14 and ejaculation for boys between 12 and 14. Girls are usually ahead of boys by about a year.

Are puberty and adolescence the same thing?

Puberty is an event within adolescence, an indication of the physical changes taking place within the body. The maturing of reproductive organs, however, is only one aspect of growing up. Adolescence refers to the long stage between the ages of about 12 and 18, when a young person matures physically and emotionally.

If sexual maturity starts with puberty, why did I get pubic hair when I was 10?

The body spends years preparing for reproduction. The process begins when the hypothalamus, a tiny gland in the brain, starts sending messages via the pituitary gland to the reproductive organs – ovaries in girls, testes in boys. These are now instructed to produce male and female hormones for the first time. But it takes about another two years for ovaries to produce oestrogen and about a year for the testes to produce testosterone. Meanwhile, the changing levels of hormones are also causing the appearance of so-called secondary features – such as pubic and facial hair and enlarged breasts and genitals.

Section two: GROWING UP

Why do my friends have hair on their bodies when I don't?

Everyone has their own biological clock. All the changes which take place during puberty, including the growth of body hair, are caused by the release of hormones. This takes place at different times and rates for each individual. So, the changes occur more quickly for some, and even in a different order. The rate of hair growth, its colour and texture also vary from person to person. The illustration shows the likely times for the development of body hair for the average girl and boy.

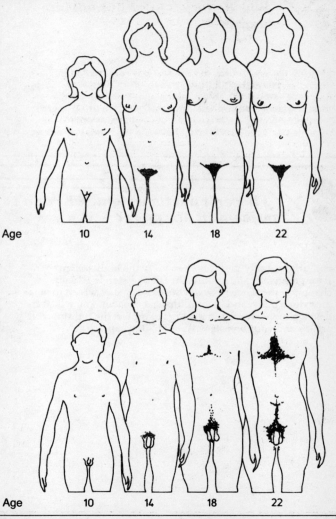

Age 10 14 18 22

Age 10 14 18 22

Section two: GROWING UP

Why do boys' voices break but not girls'?

At birth, the vocal cords of girls and boys are the same length, and in early childhood the voices of both sexes are at about the same pitch. By about the age of 10, however, boys' vocal cords are beginning to grow longer than those of girls, even though girls are often taller. As puberty approaches, boys' voices 'break', wavering between high and low notes,

I haven't put on weight. Why don't my jeans fit any more?

For girls, puberty involves changes to the body that prepare it for pregnancy and childbirth. The skeleton is actually changing: the space between the pelvic bones widen to make room for a baby, and so your hips get broader. You will also develop more fat around the hips to protect the reproductive organs and your breasts will start to develop.

until gradually the pitch settles down. Girls' voices deepen, too, but less noticeably. The vocal cords continue to grow until people are about 30 years of age.

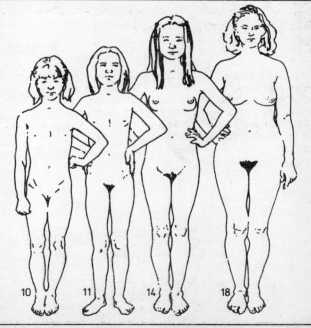

Age 10 11 14 18

Section two: GROWING UP

When does the womb reach its full size?

Before puberty, girls' reproductive organs are quite small. By 10 years of age, for instance, the ovaries are still only about one-third adult size and the uterus (womb) about half its eventual size. With sexual maturity, the uterus becomes pear-shaped, growing to about the size of its owner's fist.

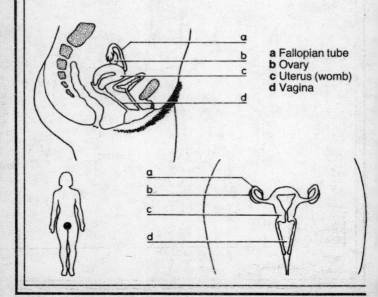

a Fallopian tube
b Ovary
c Uterus (womb)
d Vagina

When does a girl become fertile?

Girls start to have periods (begin menstruating) at about 13 years of age, but they may not become fertile for some months afterwards – perhaps up to a year. Fertility is only reached when the eggs (ova), which have been present in the ovaries since birth, begin to mature. One egg (ovum) is released each month at the point in the cycle known as ovulation.

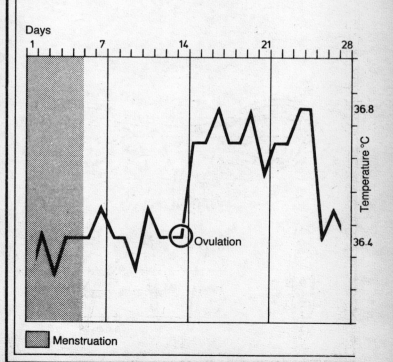

Section two: GROWING UP

How does the egg get into the womb?

At ovulation, the fringed ends of the Fallopian tubes curl round each ovary, to catch the mature ovum (egg) as it is released. The muscular walls of the Fallopian tubes are lined with millions of microscopic hairs (cilia), which help the ovum travel along its journey towards the uterus (womb).

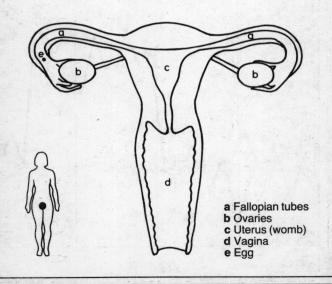

a Fallopian tubes
b Ovaries
c Uterus (womb)
d Vagina
e Egg

Why do girls have periods?

Periods are part of nature's elaborate plan for reproduction. As you can see from this illustration of the menstrual cycle, the uterus is made ready each month for pregnancy: its lining is thickened to receive a fertilized egg. If conception does not take place – the egg is not fertilized – this lining breaks down. Its cells, together with a small amount of blood, are shed in the menstrual flow (period).

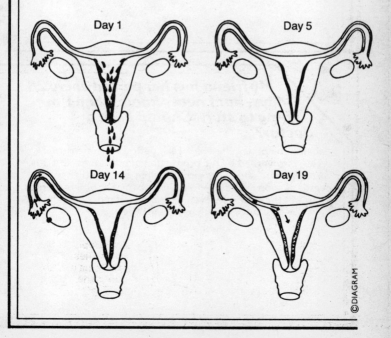

Section two: GROWING UP

Why am I the only girl in my class who hasn't started periods?

Probably the last thing you want to be is different. But the fact is that each one of us is unique. This means that your body – and everyone else's – functions at its own rate. Puberty, the beginning of menstruation, is determined by the release of hormones according to your own internal timetable, regardless of when your friends start.

My friend has her period every 28 days, but I never know when I'm going to start. Should I see a doctor?

The number of days between each period – the menstrual cycle – is governed by the production of hormones, and this varies from person to person. For some girls another cycle begins as soon as the previous one is over. For others there is a gap – or the cycle may even be completed more quickly. Very few girls have completely regular periods.

What should I do to make my periods regular?

It may be inconvenient to have irregular periods, but it is by no means abnormal. The menstrual cycle may be as short as three weeks or as long as five. It may be shorter one month that the next. If you miss too many periods, it would be a good idea to talk to your doctor. The pill is sometimes prescribed to help make periods more regular.

Regular cycle

Irregular cycle

◯ Days when ovulation may occur

Section two: GROWING UP

How can you tell when your period is going to start?

Once you have started to menstruate regularly, you will soon learn to recognize tell-tale signs in yourself which mean that the next period is on its way. No two people have all the same signs, but there are many common ones which you may experience. For instance, you may put on some weight (often because there is a slight build up of water in your body); your appetite may change; you may notice a change of texture in your skin or your hair; you may tire more easily or be more likely to get upset. These symptoms are not just 'all in the mind' – the changing level of hormones in the body can have many effects. Many girls like to jot down the dates of their periods, to remind themselves when the next one is due. This sometimes helps them to feel all right about the changes.

What is PMT?

PMT is short for premenstrual tension, the term used for the feelings of discomfort, tenseness and irritability which many girls and women get just before the period begins. It is due to a complex sequence of events to do with changing hormone levels. Often the worst effect is the fact that you tend to retain fluid just before a period, and this may lead to a slightly bloated feeling. It may also account for the irritability.

Any girl who suffers serious premenstrual symptoms, including perhaps nausea and pain, should go and see the doctor. There are ways of relieving the symptoms, and you should not have to have your life disrupted in this way each month.

Section two: GROWING UP

Is it okay to do games when I have my period?

Yes it is. This is a particularly good time to exercise, since moderate activity helps relieve cramps and the sensation of heaviness often experienced during a period. If you are bleeding a lot, it is a good idea to use a tampon and a sanitary towel for extra protection.

How can you use a tampon if you're still a virgin?

The delicate membrane known as the hymen (or maidenhead) is only a partial covering at the entrance to the vagina. There are a lot of myths relating to this small piece of tissue. The chances are that, by the time your periods begin, it will already have been broken. All it takes is vigorous exercise. In rare cases, the opening may be unusually narrow, and so it should be stretched gently. It is always best to experiment with the smallest sized tampons first.

How do I know which size tampons to use?

The size of tampon you use depends on the amount of menstrual flow, not on how big you are. 'Super' tampons absorb more fluid than 'regular' tampons. If you are using tampons for the first time, you will find it easier to start with a small size, to get used to inserting them. Some tampons have cardboard applicators to help put them in, but they all have instructions.

Tampons without applicators

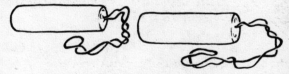

Tampons with applicators

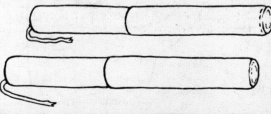

Section two: GROWING UP

I have trouble using tampons. How will I ever make love?

It is not always easy to use tampons. If you have already had difficulty inserting one in the vagina, you may become tense when you try again. One answer is to relax and find a more comfortable position so that you can follow the line of the vagina, instead of perhaps forcing a tampon against its muscular wall. At the beginning or end of a period, the vagina may be extra dry, and it will help to put a little KY jelly (not Vaseline) on the tip of the applicator.

In love-making, conditions are far more favourable. The vagina becomes lubricated naturally when you are sexually aroused and its walls expand to allow the partner's penis to enter.

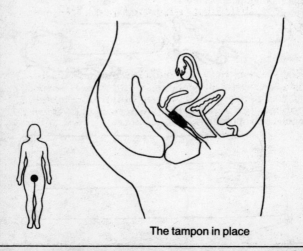

The tampon in place

Can you 'lose' a tampon?

There is no way that a tampon can be completely lost in your body because the opening of the cervix, at the far end of the vagina, is too narrow to allow it to get through into the womb. If you can't find the string by which a tampon is normally withdrawn, get yourself in a position where you can reach inside the vagina and grasp the tampon itself. If you can't get it out, you must get help, either from your mother or a doctor or nurse. You can't simply leave it inside you because it may cause an infection.

Will tampons make me ill?

Millions of women use tampons all the time with no ill-effects. The most important thing to remember is personal hygiene. Tampons should be changed every four to six hours to prevent any risk of infection, and remember to remove the last one at the end of a period.

Section two: GROWING UP

My periods have stopped and I am growing facial hair. Is something wrong?

It is common for teenagers to have irregular periods. And it is especially likely at times of severe emotional stress – if your parents are getting divorced, say, if you have to change schools, or if someone close dies. Your body may react by interrupting the normal cycle of hormones released by the glands and then the periods may stop altogether. You may also notice hair growing on your chin and neck. These are signs that your hormone balance is upset. You should see your doctor because the condition can be treated very easily. If the facial hair embarrasses you, see a professional beautician.

If I miss a period, am I pregnant?

If you have not had sexual intercourse, then certainly you are not pregnant. Especially in your teens, you may not have started to menstruate regularly. It often takes time for the complex hormone cycle to become established. But if you have had sex and miss a period, you may be pregnant, and should have a test as soon as possible.

Can all women have babies?

Women's bodies are adapted to childbearing. All the features you will become conscious of at puberty – broad hips, extra 'cushioning' around the hips and backside, powerful hormones and the development of breasts – are all geared to this purpose. However, some women have difficulty conceiving and may need medical help. Some of the causes of such difficulty are shown on the diagram.

a Blocked Fallopian tubes
b Malfunctioning ovaries
c Tilted or divided uterus
d Hostile cervical fluid
e Narrow or divided vagina
f Hymen too strong for penetration

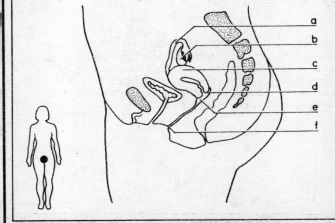

Section two: GROWING UP

What is a clitoris and where is it?

Girls may be less aware of their sexual organs than boys because their external ones are smaller and less obvious. But girls can get as much pleasure as boys from love-making, and the clitoris is usually the focal point of this pleasure. It is at the front of the vulva and covered by a little hood. Its tissues are well supplied with blood vessels and nerve endings, which make it very sensitive to touch. When it is stimulated, the clitoris swells and becomes hard.

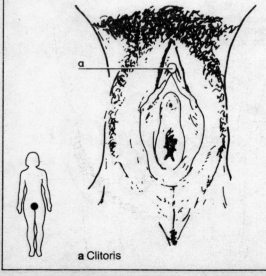

a Clitoris

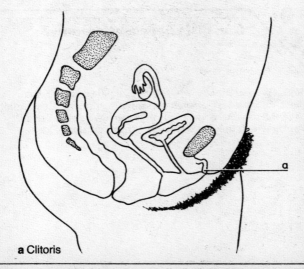

a Clitoris

Section two: GROWING UP

Why do I get wet when I think about making love?

When people become sexually aroused, their bodies begin to prepare for intercourse. The man has an erection; in women the glands in the wall of the vagina produce a lubricating fluid to make entry of the penis easier and more comfortable for both partners. This fluid also moistens the vulva on the outside and increases the pleasure you get from being touched.

Can girls have wet dreams?

Boys have wet dreams when they ejaculate semen in their sleep, due to a sexy or even a frightening dream. Girls cannot have wet dreams as such, but they can have a sexy dream during which they become aroused and lubricate.

Vaginal deodorants make me itch. Do I need to use them?

The need for vaginal deodorants, or floral-scented tampons or perfumed powder is a myth. There is no substitute for cleanliness. If you feel self-conscious about the smell of your body when it is clean, remember that it is part of your sexual attractiveness. The skin around the vagina is very sensitive. If you use a deodorant or perfume, it could cause problems like burning or itching.

One of my breasts seems to be growing larger than the other. What's wrong?

You may be surprised to know that the left and right sides of your body are neither the same size nor the same shape. This lack of symmetry is normal, even the two profiles of your face are different. So, you can expect your breasts to grow at different rates and to vary a little in shape. You are probably the only one who notices the difference.

Section two: GROWING UP

My breasts are too small. Can't I do something to make them grow?

Your breasts are still growing and changing, even if you are not satisfied with the way they look right now. There is nothing you can do to hasten their growth, and anyone who tries to sell you creams guaranteed to increase breast size is taking your money under false pretences. Exercise is no help either, since there are no muscles in the breast tissue itself.

Can you have a baby if you have small breasts?

It may be of concern to you, but the size of your breasts makes no difference when you become pregnant. As you mature sexually, the glands and ducts that will produce and deliver milk become enlarged, but it is the pads of fat between the glands that determine how big your breasts are. During pregnancy, the glands become larger to prepare for lactation (production of milk), and so your breasts swell.

If I don't wear a bra, will I be able to breastfeed when I have a baby?

You wear a bra mostly for your own comfort. Breasts do not have muscles but are supported by strong ligaments. When you are pregnant and your breasts become enlarged, you will need the support of a good bra.

What colour should my nipples be?

The nipples are surrounded by a circular area of skin called the areola. This, along with the nipple, usually darkens at puberty; it continues to change colour and shape slightly throughout life. Areolae and nipples vary in size and colour: it is just as normal for them to be small and pink as large and brown.

Section two: GROWING UP

My nipples are flat. Is there something wrong with them?

Most of the time nipples are flat and soft. But when the breasts are stimulated – if stroked or if you stand under a cold shower – tiny muscles at the base of each nipple make them erect and firm.

When should you start checking your breasts for lumps?

Women check their breasts for any changes, including lumps (most of which prove to be harmless). Although cysts or tumours of the breast do not usually develop until you are older, it is a good idea to learn breast self-examination early on and to make it a life-long routine. Your doctor or a nurse can show you the simple recommended procedure.

Can men get breast cancer?

Yes they can, but it is very rare indeed, far less of a risk in men than in women.

Can men's breasts produce milk?

No, they can't because they lack the milk-producing glands and ducts of the female.

Section two: GROWING UP

My penis looks so small. Will I be able to have sex?

Stories about penis size are a bit like fishermen's tales: they tend to get bigger in the telling. In fact, most penises are more or less the same size when erect (16.5 cm or so), and it is rubbish to claim that the bigger the penis, the better the lover. Measured from base to tip along its upper surface, the limp penis varies from just under 9 cm to a little over 10 cm, giving an average length of 9.5 cm. But what many people don't realise is that a penis which is smallish when limp may more than double its size on erection, while a big one may only increase by about 75 per cent. Another fallacy is: the bigger the man, the bigger the penis. Penis size has nothing to do with overall body size or big muscles. There is no appreciable difference in penis size between ethnic groups.

How can I make my penis bigger?

You can't and anyway you don't need to. There is no safe way of permanently increasing the size of the penis, and any creams or devices which claim to do this are an outright con. Your penis may look small to you, but it probably isn't; and in any case it will enlarge to a perfectly adequate length on

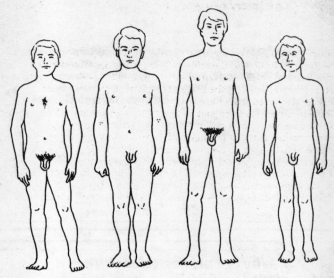

Four normal boys of the same age

arousal. Any penis tends to look small to its owner, viewed from above. Why not try looking at yourself full frontal, facing a mirror? You'll get a much better impression.

Section two: GROWING UP

Are the testicles as important as the penis?

Yes, they are, because without them you couldn't perform or even develop sexually. The testicles (or testes), contained in a pouch called the scrotum, have two important functions: they produce chemicals known as the sex hormones which help control your growth and development to manhood; and they manufacture sperm.

Why are my testicles different sizes?

It is true to say that two testicles are almost never the same. One (mostly the left) hangs lower than the other. But, of course, they will vary in appearance depending on the weather and what you're up to at any given moment. The reason they hang outside the body at all is that sperm are best produced at 1° to 2°C lower than the normal body temperature. So, usually the testicles hang clear, but in cold weather (or if you happen to be swimming in cold water) they tend to be drawn up closer to the body for warmth. The scrotum is raised, too, when you get sexually excited.

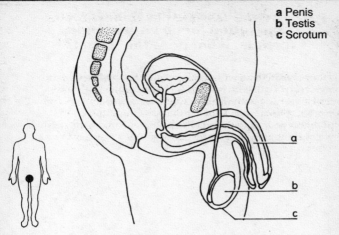

a Penis
b Testis
c Scrotum

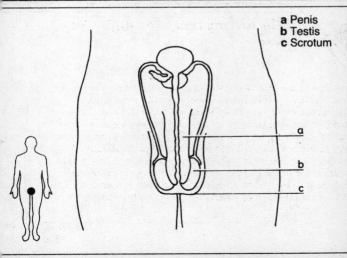

a Penis
b Testis
c Scrotum

Section two: GROWING UP

My little brother is having an operation for an undescended testicle. What does that mean?

Before birth, the testes develop inside the body and then descend into the scrotum. In some cases, one testicle is still inside the body. This problem is not uncommon, but, left untreated, it can increase the risk of infertility and, sometimes, lead to cancer after puberty. Fortunately, there is a simple operation to correct undescended testicles in small boys.

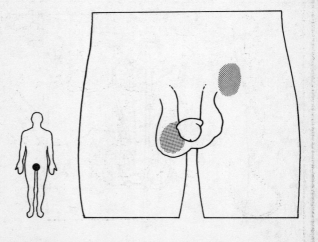

Where do sperms come from?

Sperm cells are usually just called sperm (**a**). They are very small and are produced in coiled tubules within the testes (**b**). They mature in a long tube, the epididymis (**c**), which lies over the testis and are carried along a duct known as the vas deferens (**d**) to the seminal vesicles (**e**) for storage. From here, they are released in the milky-white fluid called semen, produced in the prostate gland (**f**), which is discharged from the tip of the penis (**g**).

a Sperm shown greatly magnified

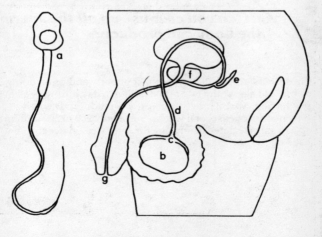

Section two: GROWING UP

How much sperm should come out when you come?

Most healthy males produce about a teaspoonful of semen when they come. But when you remember that each tiny droplet of semen contains literally tens of thousands of sperm, then it is obvious that the quantity lost at each ejaculation (when you come) runs into many millions, sometimes as much as 300 million at one time. Yet, small as it is, any one of these sperms may succeed in fertilizing the egg and starting a pregnancy.

Can you ever use up all the sperm the body can produce?

The testes start producing sperm at puberty and go on doing so into old age, at the rate of 500 million a day during peak production. Sperm move from testis to epididymis where they mature over several weeks. Since only 200 to 300 million sperm are ejaculated at any one time, they could never all be used up.

What happens to the sperm that aren't used up?

Sperm that aren't used up, or ejaculated, are eventually absorbed in the body fluids and carried away for disposal, just like other wastes.

Do all men ejaculate?

No, there are physical and psychological reasons why some men are unable to ejaculate. In their case, the unused sperms just disintegrate and are absorbed harmlessly into the body.

Section two: GROWING UP

Can you ejaculate without an erection?

No, not really. The intense feelings which accompany sexual arousal and an erection usually provide the signals needed, too, for ejaculation. In the first stage of arousal, the excitement phase (**1**), blood flows into the spongy tissues of the penis, making it start to go erect. In the plateau phase (**2**) the head of the penis and the testicles may become larger. The testicles are drawn up closer to the body in order to aid ejaculation. In the orgasmic phase (**3**), sperm mix with semen to form the ejaculate, and this is forced along the urethra to emerge usually in a series of spurts. In the resolution phase, after orgasm, the penis quickly goes limp (**4**).

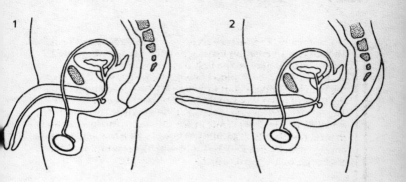

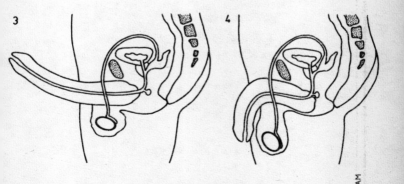

Section two: GROWING UP

How old do you have to be to have an erection?

You are never too young or too old. Baby boys can have their first erection soon after birth, and men can remain sexually active well into old age.

The penis contains three spongy erectile cylinders which run along the length of the shaft. These are richly supplied with blood vessels. All sorts of stimuli can cause an erection, but this happens especially when the highly sensitive glans and corona (the head of the penis and its encircling ridge) are touched. Compartments in the spongy cylinders begin to fill with blood and the penis stiffens and increases in thickness and length.

It's very embarrassing to feel myself getting an erection when there are other people around. What can I do to stop it?

Once you have reached puberty, you may often have erections, even at the most unexpected and awkward moments. Not only the sight – or thought – of a girl, but intense emotions like anger or fear and even strenuous physical exercise may give you an erection. You can't hide your natural reaction, but you can distract yourself by thinking of something that takes your mind off it.

I don't remember having a sexy dream, so why were my pyjamas wet when I woke up?

Everyone has dreams throughout the night, and dreaming about sex is something we all do. But remembering even one dream is an event. With the onset of puberty, sexy dreams often stimulate an erection and ejaculation – a wet dream. Frightening dreams can have the same effect. This does not mean you are a sex maniac, and the wet dreams usually tail off of their own accord.

Section two: GROWING UP

Do wet dreams hurt?

On the contrary, they are liable to produce a pleasurable sensation if you are aware of them in your sleep.

I'm worried in case I have a wet dream when I'm staying at my grandma's and she finds out. How can I stop having them?

Wet dreams are a sign that you are normal. While there is no way to control what you dream at night, you may reduce the chance of nocturnal emission by masturbating before you go to sleep. It may also help if you remember that grandmothers are married and have raised a family, too.

Do semen and pee ever get mixed together since they both come out of the same place?

Never, and there is no risk to you or to anyone you might take as a sexual partner from the fact that they share the same channel. This is because males can't urinate and ejaculate (come) at the same time. Semen never comes out when you pee and there is a special valve which automatically shuts off urine when the penis is erect. On arousal, the male sex glands leak a clear, colourless fluid which neutralizes any residue of urine in the urethra before the semen comes along. This is not urine.

My breasts are getting bigger. Has something gone wrong?

Not at all. A slight swelling of the breasts is only a temporary (if embarrassing) development that about half of all boys have to put up with during puberty.

3

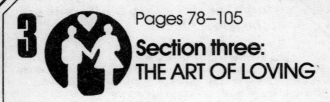

Pages 78–105

Section three:
THE ART OF LOVING

- Does everyone masturbate? 80
- Is masturbation good for you? 80
- Is masturbation bad for you? 81
- Can you masturbate too much? 81
- How do girls masturbate? 82
- How do boys masturbate? 82
- What are erogenous zones? 83
- What gives boys erections? 84
- Is a girl's nipples going hard like a boy getting an erection, or is it different? 84
- Why does petting make my testicles ache? 85
- Can sex hurt? 86
- Will I enjoy sex the first time I have it? 86
- Do people always like sex or do they get bored? 87
- How long does sex last? 87
- How do you know if you've had an orgasm? 88
- I've had sex with my boyfriend but I don't think I've had an orgasm. Why can't I come? 89
- Does everyone have orgasms? 90
- Who can have more orgasms, men or boys? 91
- Who can have more orgasms, men or women? 91
- Do you come faster from oral sex than from ordinary sex? 92
- I don't like the idea of oral sex. Am I normal? 92
- A boy I know says he can come six times in a row. Is he telling the truth? 93
- When I tried to have sex I came too soon. Will I ever get it right? 93
- Can you have sex without an erection? 94

- I tried to make love to my girlfriend and my penis went limp. Am I impotent? **95**
- What does impotent mean? **96**
- Is impotence the same as sterility? **96**
- My girlfriend said she wasn't ready to make love, but I already had an erection. Was she just trying to tell me she didn't want to? **97**
- Can a girl have sex during her period? What do you do about the blood? **98**
- People were sniggering in class the other day when the answer to a question was 69, but they wouldn't tell me why. Can you explain? **98**
- Can having sex make you ill? **99**
- How often should you have sex? **100**
- What's a good lover? **100**
- How do you tell if other people are good lovers? **101**
- How do you get to be a good lover? **101**
- Are you a better lover if you haven't been circumcised? **102**
- Does alcohol make you sexy? **102**
- If I go home after having sex, will my parents be able to tell? **104**
- How did the missionary position get its name? **104**
- What's a love bite? **105**

Section three: THE ART OF LOVING

Does everyone masturbate?

Children of both sexes often learn at a very early age that they can give themselves physical pleasure by touching or rubbing something against their genitals. Once you have reached puberty, hormones produced in the ovaries or testicles contribute to a new and growing awareness of your own sexuality and that of others. You may find that masturbation helps relieve some of the sexual tension that is an inevitable part of growing up. People used to believe that girls did not masturbate, but this is not true. Both girls and boys masturbate and some people never do. Boys generally masturbate more than girls possibly because the penis is more accessible and they are more used to touching it.

Is masturbation good for you?

Masturbation is usually the first and best way for young people to learn about their new identity as sexually responsive human beings. The attitude that good children – especially girls – remained unaware of sex until they were married has given way to the understanding that sex is normal and healthy and that it is good to explore your body and learn about your own sexuality in this way.

Is masturbation bad for you?

The old idea that masturbation is harmful – that it stunts your growth, turns you blind or even drives you insane – is now entirely discredited, and many people of both sexes practise it to some extent throughout their lives. The only thing about masturbation which is in any way damaging or bad is other people's negative attitudes to it, which may induce guilt feelings in young people for no good reason.

Can you masturbate too much?

It is possible for masturbation to become compulsive. So, while it won't hurt you, it can disturb your life like any compulsion. Some people – boys in particular – tend to masturbate more if they are worried about something. This is not harmful in itself, but, of course, it won't solve your problems.

Section three: THE ART OF LOVING

How do girls masturbate?

Girls and women masturbate mostly with their hands, rubbing against the sensitive clitoris at the top of the vulva. Or they may use a firmer action over the whole vulva, sometimes using one or more fingers to enter the vagina and mimic the rhythmic movements of intercourse.

How do boys masturbate?

A boy masturbates by first of all stroking the sensitive head of the penis to stimulate an erection. As the penis stiffens, he makes a fist of one hand and, starting at the base, moves the hand backwards and forwards along the length of the penis. The movement becomes faster and faster as the climax approaches. Afterwards, when he has ejaculated, the penis quickly becomes limp.

What are erogenous zones?

Certain parts of the body are very sensitive to touch. When these so-called erogenous zones are stroked or licked, the boy or girl becomes sexually aroused. The most responsive regions are the genitals, the penis and the clitoris. But many people are aroused (get turned on) when other parts of the body are touched, especially the inside of the mouth, the earlobes, nipples, the insides of the thighs and buttocks. The diagram shows the primary (**A**) and most usual secondary (**B**) erogenous zones. As two people come to know and love each other, they discover many extra-responsive places in themselves and their partners.

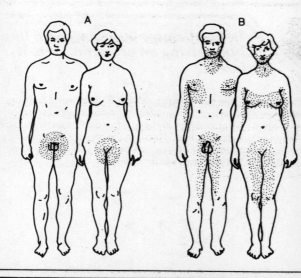

Section three: THE ART OF LOVING

What gives boys erections?

Various stimuli can bring on an erection, including fear, but most often, it is some kind of sexual signal which causes the penis to become erect. Sometimes it is caused by an erotic photograph or by the sight of a pretty girl; sometimes just the thought of a girl or of love-making is enough to make it happen.

What actually happens is that, when a boy gets excited, the ring of muscle at the base of the penis tightens so that blood can flow into it but not out (as it would otherwise do at a steady rate). This makes the penis swell and harden. Afterwards, when the boy has ejaculated, the muscle relaxes, the blood flow returns to normal and the penis goes limp.

Is a girl's nipples going hard like a boy getting an erection, or is it different?

It isn't exactly the same thing, although the nipples are very sensitive and tend to harden and stand out as a girl starts to get excited. What is closer in the girl to a boy's erection is the change in the clitoris. For it, too – the most sensitive part of the female sex organs – swells and becomes engorged with blood when the girl becomes aroused.

Why does petting make my testicles ache?

As a boy becomes sexually aroused and has an erection, the scrotum tenses and swells; the testicles also become enlarged and are drawn up closer to the body. If this stage of sexual tension continues, the testicles almost double in size. If orgasm follows, the testicles will return to their normal size and position fairly rapidly. If the boy does not come and the swelling is not relieved, he will feel a deep ache in the groin, sometimes known as 'lover's balls'. It is not dangerous and will soon disappear.

Not aroused

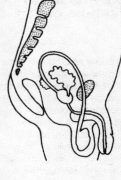

Aroused

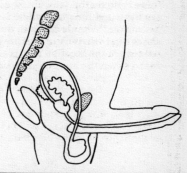

Section three: THE ART OF LOVING

Can sex hurt?

Many girls are afraid that having sex will hurt, especially for the first time. While there may be a brief twinge of pain when the penis first enters a virgin's vagina (if the hymen is still intact), penetration should not be painful after that. It is very important for the girl to be fully aroused so that the vagina is well lubricated. If the vagina is dry, sex can be unpleasant and painful, and the walls of the vagina can become sore. People in love want to be sensitive to the feelings and needs of their partners and make sex free from fear.

Will I enjoy sex the first time I have it?

There is no reason why you shouldn't enjoy sex the first time you have it. But equally, there is nothing magic about sex that makes it wonderful from the start. If you are in the back seat of a car where your legs are cramped, you are afraid of getting caught, worried in case they notice something different when you get home, not really sure how you feel about your partner, afraid of getting pregnant, you should not be surprised if sex doesn't seem all it's cracked up to be. On the other hand, two people who care a great deal for each other (and already respond to each other's needs) can be pretty confident that sex will be an important part of their relationship from the beginning.

Do people always like sex or do they get bored?

It is possible to enjoy sex on a purely sensual or physical level. Most people discover (if they don't know already) the emotional side of sex: the way a couple feel closer and more open to each other after making love, and the way sex becomes part of a private language between two lovers. Sex only becomes boring when people become bored with each other.

How long does sex last?

Sex can last as long as you want it to. If you look at it just in terms of the main chance, orgasm as such can be over in about 10 seconds – for the man at least. But, as you will come to realize, there is much more to love-making than intercourse.

Section three: THE ART OF LOVING

How do you know if you've had an orgasm?

Boys know that they have had an orgasm because they have ejaculated. The sensation of intense pleasure comes as the semen is forced out by powerful contractions of muscles and tissues in and around the penis. This is accompanied by rapid breathing and a racing heart-beat as the tension builds up and is then released. Often, the boy will perspire and may even break out in a measles-like 'sex flush'.

The focal point of orgasm in women, whether they come during intercourse, petting or masturbation, is the clitoris. As the vulva is stimulated, the sensation of pleasure gradually increases. The clitoris swells, and the vagina produces its lubricant fluid. The girl breathes more rapidly, and her heart-beat races as she reaches a climax with an intensity of feeling which spreads throughout the body. She may be aware of short, involuntary spasms in the vagina.

Orgasm leaves both boys and girls feeling satisfied, intimate and sleepy.

I've had sex with my boyfriend but I don't think I've had an orgasm. Why can't I come?

It is impossible to describe adequately the strength of feelings experienced with orgasm because they can vary in intensity. But what you should look for is a pleasurable sensation that builds up over time. Your body becomes tense, then with orgasm you experience a relaxation and warmth throughout the body.

A common reason why girls have difficulty in coming is that having an orgasm is something they have to learn. They have to find out for themselves how their body responds to stimuli and, if necessary, show their sex partner how it works. Girls enjoy an interval of foreplay which allows them to be sexually stimulated and aroused. They also need to feel free from anxiety or guilt feeling, to experience love-making to the full.

Section three: THE ART OF LOVING

Does everyone have orgasms?

No, they don't, at least not all the time. Men experience orgasms more than women. Unless they are impotent, or temporarily unable to keep an erection, due perhaps to drink or drugs, they are almost bound to come once the arousal mechanism is set in motion. With women, the process is not so simple and direct, and some women have never experienced orgasm, often because they haven't had enough stimulation.

Ideally, partners should work towards each other's satisfaction and enjoyment of love-making, but you can enjoy sex without necessarily coming every time and this should not be regarded as a failure. The important thing is to take the time your body needs to enjoy sex whether you have an orgasm or not.

Who can have more orgasms, men or boys?

Boys can come more often than men can: as they grow up boys find that they have to wait longer between each erection. The number of orgasms has little to do with the ability to be a good lover. Research has established that, when orgasm is less frequent, the volume of seminal fluid building up in the reproductive organs makes it a more intense experience.

Who can have more orgasms, men or women?

Some girls find they can have a series of orgasms with only a few seconds between each one but men have to wait for another erection. However, most people are perfectly satisfied just having one orgasm.

Section three: THE ART OF LOVING

Do you come faster from oral sex than from ordinary sex?

It depends entirely on your likes and dislikes and on those of your partner as well. If both partners enjoy oral sex, and can practise it without inhibition, it is possible to make each other come very quickly this way. But if one or other partner is a bit reluctant to practise oral sex, it could be rather frustrating.

I don't like the idea of oral sex. Am I normal?

Of course you are. By no means everyone enjoys oral sex. It is very commonly practised, but if you don't even like the idea of it, don't let yourself be blackmailed or otherwise pressurized into it against your will.

A boy I know says he can come six times in a row. Is he telling the truth?

He could be, but did he tell you how long he had to wait between erections? The younger you are, the more often you can come, and around the onset of puberty this can be as frequent as every few minutes. As you mature sexually, you will find that the resting time between erections increases.

When I tried to have sex I came too soon. Will I ever get it right?

We often find that reality falls far short of our fantasies, and boys who imagine themselves as great lovers get a shock when their early efforts suffer from bad timing. Premature ejaculation (coming too soon) is a common problem, especially before boys realize that girls may take much longer to get turned on than they do. One solution is for the couple to concentrate on foreplay, an important part of love-making. If the boy doesn't have to wait too long between erections, he can masturbate first; then the couple can give each other a lot of sexual pleasure with their hands and mouths until he is ready to have another erection. The best solution, however, is to work at achieving a stable and satisfying relationship.

Section three: THE ART OF LOVING

Can you have sex without an erection?

A boy will not be able to put his limp penis inside a girl's vagina because the muscular vaginal walls require fairly firm pressure in order to be spread apart. If you have already come once and want to continue love-making before you have another erection, you can use this time to explore each other's bodies.

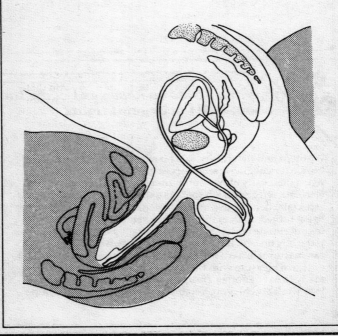

I tried making love to my girlfriend and my penis went limp. Am I impotent?

If you have ever had an erection, masturbated successfully or had a wet dream, you are certainly not impotent. You are no less a man just because you failed to make it once, although you may feel inadequate. Very few men suffer from impotence, where they are incapable of having an erection and keeping it. On the other hand, your experience is one suffered by almost all boys and men at some time. Except for injury to the sex organs, the cause of impotence is psychological, not physical. That is not to say, however, that the problem and the anguish of impotence are not real. The good news is you and your partner can do something about it, because it can be overcome.

Successful love-making is a complex process. It is not about how good I am, but how good *we* are. You can be turned off by the wrong partner, or by having sex under difficult circumstances (like expecting your parents to come home any minute). If your upbringing or your own attitudes make you feel that sex is wrong or 'dirty', you may find that you can't keep an erection. If your partner feels that you are insensitive to her needs, she may be turned off, and that's catching. Often, inability to make love is caused by a fear of being a failure. The more you worry about your performance, the harder it becomes.

So, relax. With patience and consideration on both sides, the problem should sort itself out.

Section three: THE ART OF LOVING

What does impotent mean?

A man who is unable to have an erection or to maintain it long enough to have sex is impotent. This is very uncommon in boys. Occasionally, the cause of impotence is physical. Sex may be difficult for handicapped people, and drugs and alcohol can make a boy temporarily impotent. In most instances, impotence is related to psychological problems. If a boy has had a bad experience with a girl, he may not be able to have an erection the next time he tries to have sex.

Is impotence the same as sterility?

No. The reason that people who are sterile cannot become parents is that their reproductive organs do not produce sperms or eggs for fertilization. The causes of sterility in women are much more complicated than they are in men as the sperm fertilizes the egg inside the woman's body, and this may be prevented in a number of ways. Men who are impotent are not sterile unless they do not produce sperm, but because they are unable to penetrate, they cannot take part in the natural conception process. Equally, sterile men are not necessarily impotent.

My girlfriend said she wasn't ready to make love, but I already had an erection. Was she just trying to tell me she didn't want to?

Girls are no different from boys in having a deep, intense need for sex. Where the two differ are in their expressions of this need. Traditionally, our society has demanded that boys demonstrate their strong adolescent sexuality while girls suppress theirs, and guilt or shame often prevent people from expressing their true feelings. The stimuli and the timing of sexual arousal also differ between the sexes. In general, boys get turned on more quickly, for example, in response to sexy pictures or to fondling their girlfriends' breasts. Girls usually take longer to become fully aroused – ready for intercourse – and, for them, the prolonged stimulation of being cuddled, kissed and stroked are essential parts of love-making.

Can a girl have sex during her period? What do you do about the blood?

There is no reason why a girl shouldn't have sex while she is menstruating if she chooses. In fact, many girls feel sexier during a period than at ovulation, the time of greatest fertility. If a girl is worried about the menstrual flow, she can use a diaphragm to contain the blood temporarily. It is also an idea to put a thick towel beneath you to prevent accidental staining.

Sometimes, at this point in the cycle, the vagina and cervix are a bit painful. So, it's a good idea for the couple to find a position which allows the girl to control the depth of penetration during intercourse.

People were sniggering in class the other day when the answer to a question was 69, but they wouldn't tell me why. Can you explain?

Sixty-nine, also known as *soixante-neuf* in French, is a slang term for oral sex, where the girl takes the boy's penis in her mouth while the boy touches the girl's vulva with his tongue. It is called this because the position the two partners get into resembles the figures 69.

Can having sex make you ill?

Sex can be either good or bad for you: good when you have a caring, responsible relationship that makes you want only good things for your partner; bad when one or both of you is being hurt in some way. Girls still tend to suffer from the attitude that, for them, sex before marriage is wrong, and they may have to decide whether to have sex in the face of disapproving authorities. So it is tempting to dismiss reports that link early, frequent sex with illness as nothing more than part of another moral campaign.

For some years now, doctors have been worried by a rise in the incidence of cancer of the cervix among young women, and they have made a connection between this disease and an early, active sex life. Recent research has suggested that cancer of the cervix is, in fact, a sexually transmitted disease (STD) caused by the same virus that causes genital warts. Men who have had many sex partners may be responsible for passing the disease to each woman with whom they have intercourse. It seems to be true that the more partners a man has, the more likelihood there is of damage to the cervix which may lead to cancer. Frequent sex with many partners also increases the risk of other STDs and urinary infections for both sexes and vaginitis for women.

The best defence, aside from changing your lifestyle, is to use a barrier method of contraception. The diaphragm or the condom plus a spermicide does shield the cervix, offering some protection. It is also important for the girl to be examined regularly, so that any change in the cervix can be treated before it becomes a serious problem.

Section three: THE ART OF LOVING

How often should you have sex?

There is no rule-book for love-making. When, where and how you have sex and how often depends entirely on the way you and your partner feel.

What's a good lover?

Being a good lover has everything to do with sensitivity to the needs and responses of your partner and a willingness to communicate with each other about those needs. Experience in love-making is important; good lovers learn from their partners. But, even between two people after many years of marriage, there is no sure formula for success because human beings are changing all the time.

How do you tell if other people are good lovers?

Not by the size of their breasts or the bulge at the front of their jeans. The idea that there is some sort of lover's proficiency badge is wishful thinking, largely because the quality of your love-making depends not least on the quality of your relationship.

How do you get to be a good lover?

Plenty of books describe varieties of sexual techniques if you feel that you and your partner need more ideas. So long as you trust each other and talk to each other and don't feel guilty, you can learn countless different ways to increase each other's pleasure and satisfaction.

Section three: THE ART OF LOVING

Are you a better lover if you haven't been circumcised?

People often think that men who've been circumcised cannot control ejaculation as well as men who have not had the foreskin removed. But this is yet another myth. During an erection, the foreskin usually draws back from the sensitive glans (the head of the penis) so at this stage it is hard to tell if someone has been circumcised (**A**) or not (**B**). Circumcision, a simple procedure to remove the foreskin (prepuce), can be done at any age and is often performed on new-borns for religious reasons; or, in many hospitals, baby boys are circumcised soon after birth for reasons of hygiene. If you still have a foreskin, it is important to wash carefully beneath it to avoid infection.

Does alcohol make you sexy?

You may feel sexy when you've had a few drinks, but alcohol isn't making you a better lover, it's simply lowering your inhibitions. After you've had one too many, the chances are you won't be able to have intercourse at all.

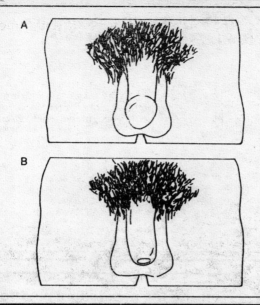

Section three: THE ART OF LOVING

If I go home after having sex, will my parents be able to tell?

Having sex does not leave any visible marks (apart from love bites perhaps). If you have a satisfying sexual relationship, you will inevitably look happier and more contented. If you are feeling guilty and dread getting caught, your behaviour may give you away.

How did the missionary position get its name?

It is believed that this intriguing phrase was coined by Polynesians when they first discovered how European missionaries had sex – lying down, face to face, with the man on top. In those days sex was still regarded as a sinful necessity – in European society, if not among the Polynesians – and this position was somehow the least objectionable way of having intercourse.

What's a love bite?

A love bite isn't really a bite. It is the mark made by a kiss where the partner sucks on a small area of skin. Prolonged suction bruises the tiny blood vessels lying just beneath the surface of the skin, leaving a typically round, red mark.

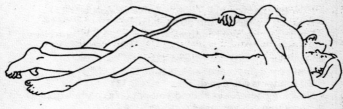

4

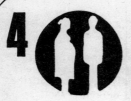

Pages 106–143

Section four:
THE QUESTION OF PREGNANCY

- Can you have a baby if you've never had intercourse? **108**
- Can you get pregnant the first time you make love? **109**
- Can you get pregnant if you have sex standing up? **109**
- Can you get pregnant if you don't have an orgasm? **110**
- Can oral sex make you pregnant? **112**
- Can anal sex make you pregnant? **112**
- Can you get pregnant if you have sex during your period? **113**
- If you haven't got contraceptives, is there any way you can have sex without risking pregnancy? **113**
- Can you use tampons as contraceptives? **114**
- What is a safe period? **114**
- If your periods are irregular, is there a form of natural birth control you can use? **116**
- Why are people taught about contraception before they're ready to have sex? **117**
- What can they tell from an internal examination? **118**
- How do I know which contraceptive works best? **120**
- What's a smear test and do I need one? **121**
- I don't like buying condoms at the chemists. Where else can I get them? **121**
- Should a girl carry condoms? **122**
- Don't condoms make sex less fun? **122**
- Do condoms come in different sizes? **123**
- How long before sex should you put on a condom? **123**
- How often can you use a condom? **124**
- Are condoms really safe? **124**
- How long do sperm live? **126**

- What does a spermicide do? **126**
- I want to have sex, but I'm too frightened to go and get contraceptives. My friend says she will let me use her diaphragm. Is this safe? **127**
- My girlfriend has a diaphragm but it looks enormous. How does she get it in? **128**
- Can you have sex more than once with the diaphragm inside you, or do you have to take it out after each time? **129**
- How does an IUD work? **130**
- Is it true that IUDs can move around your body? **131**
- Can you use tampons if you've got an IUD? **131**
- Does using contraceptives stop your periods? **132**
- Why are there so many names for the pill? Are they all the same? **132**
- Why do you have to go to the doctor if you want to go on the pill? Why can't you just go to the chemists? **133**
- How does the pill work? Does it kill sperm? **133**
- Can you get addicted to the pill? Can it make you high or turn you on? **134**
- Is it possible to get pregnant on the pill? **134**
- How many times can you miss taking the pill and know that you're still safe? **135**
- How is the mini-pill different from the pill? **135**
- What is the 'morning after' pill? **136**
- Is there an injection that stops you getting pregnant? **136**
- Why don't they have a pill for boys? **137**
- I don't fancy spending years messing around with contraceptives. Can't I be sterilized and have it reversed later? **137**
- My father has had a vasectomy. Does this mean he can't make love any more? **138**
- My aunt has had her tubes tied. What does this mean? **139**
- If you have sex and don't use a contraceptive, is there anything you can use afterwards to stop yourself getting pregnant? **140**
- How long should you wait to find out if you're pregnant? **141**
- I think I might be pregnant. What should I do? **142**
- Are home pregnancy tests reliable, or should you go to a doctor? **142**
- Do you have to tell your parents if you need an abortion? **143**
- I'm pregnant and my mother wants me to have an abortion, but I want to keep the baby. What can I do? **143**

Section four: THE QUESTION OF PREGNANCY

Can you have a baby if you've never had intercourse?

If live sperm come into contact with the vulva, there is no reason why they cannot enter the vagina and swim up through the cervix to the uterus (womb). Strictly speaking, a girl can still be a virgin and become pregnant, although this rarely happens. The time when you have to be careful is when your partner has an orgasm and ejaculates onto the vulva. In case semen does come into contact with your sex organs, the best thing to do is to wash yourself gently but thoroughly, but there is no guarantee that washing will prevent pregnancy.

Can you get pregnant the first time you make love?

You can. There are many tales about avoiding getting pregnant, and it is pretty safe to say that none of them is true. Any time you have intercourse – even the first time – you run the risk of getting pregnant if you don't use contraceptives.

Can you get pregnant if you have sex standing up?

There is no position which prevents conception. It doesn't matter what you and your partner were doing, or if you were fully clothed, when sperm were ejaculated into the vagina. The sperm will always swim up towards the uterus. If a mature egg is released by the ovaries within a day or two, it will probably be fertilized.

Section four: THE QUESTION OF PREGNANCY

Can you get pregnant if you don't have an orgasm?

Yes, pregnancy is always a possibility if you have intercourse. Sexual arousal is an essential part of enjoyable sex, partly because at this stage the vagina is preparing for penetration by expanding and producing lubricating fluid. During the next stage of love-making, called the plateau phase, the lower end of the vagina grips the penis while the end near the cervix becomes enlarged (this is where semen will collect after your partner has ejaculated), and the uterus and cervix are drawn upwards. Studies have shown that the plateau phase provides the best condition for fertilization. If you reach orgasm, you will experience rippling contractions along the vaginal muscles gripping the penis, but this in itself does not increase your chances of conceiving.

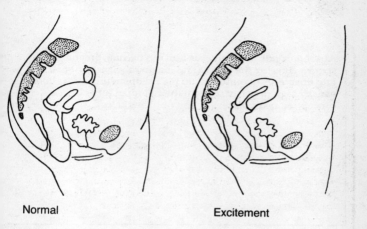

Normal

Excitement

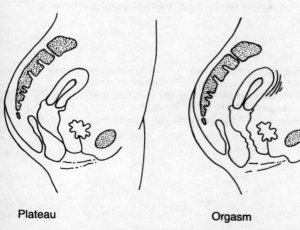

Plateau

Orgasm

Section four: THE QUESTION OF PREGNANCY

Can oral sex make you pregnant?

Absolutely not. The only way you can become pregnant is by sperms entering the vagina and making their way from there into the uterus (womb) and up the Fallopian tubes. It is here, usually high in one or other of the Fallopian tubes, that conception takes place: a sperm fertilizes an egg.

Can anal sex make you pregnant?

Not in the ordinary way, but the risk of semen anywhere near the sex organs making their way into the vagina is there. It would only take a droplet of semen, containing thousands of sperms, to enter the vagina and the risk of pregnancy would be as real as if you'd had intercourse in the usual way.

Can you get pregnant if you have sex during your period?

Ovulation can occur at any time. If a mature egg happens to be released from the ovary while you are menstruating, then you could possibly become pregnant if you have sex without using contraceptives.

If you haven't got contraceptives, is there any way you can have sex without risking pregnancy?

There is always a likelihood of pregnancy if you have penetration without the protection of contraceptives. The only alternatives are to postpone love-making until you have contraceptives to use, or to seek ways of giving each other sexual satisfaction without 'going all the way'.

Section four: THE QUESTION OF PREGNANCY

Can you use tampons as contraceptives?

No, the only thing that tampons can prevent is full penetration because there simply isn't room inside the vagina for a tampon and an erect penis. Tampons do not seal off the cervix, so any sperm that get past can still get to the uterus and fertilize an egg.

What is a safe period?

Some people prefer not to use artificial contraception, but choose instead to make love only at the times in the menstrual cycle when a woman is least likely to become pregnant. This means avoiding intercourse for about four or five days before and after ovulation (see chart). But, since it is impossible to know in advance precisely when ovulation will take place, these so-called 'safe' periods are not wholly safe, only slightly less risky than other times of the month.

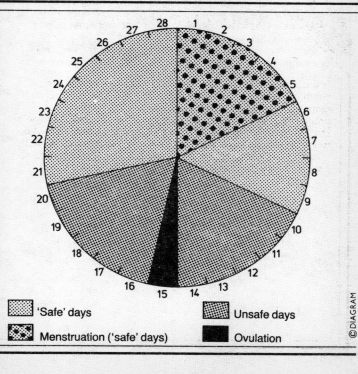

- 'Safe' days
- Unsafe days
- Menstruation ('safe' days)
- Ovulation

Section four: THE QUESTION OF PREGNANCY

> *If your periods are irregular, is there a form of natural birth control that you can use?*

Natural birth control depends on a regular cycle and rhythm methods are not usually a good form of contraception for girls because they depend for success on times of abstinence (when both partners do not make love). Married couples can build this into their relationship, but it requires a great deal of patience and self-control, and even then it is not very reliable.

Some women use a temperature cycle. The temperature is taken every day, and, when the body heat rises by about half a degree C, they know that they have ovulated. They must then wait several days before making love and must stop again when their periods start.

Another method is based on the changes in the vaginal discharge throughout the menstrual cycle. This requires very careful attention and is rather imprecise.

Why are people taught about contraception before they're ready to have sex?

Contraception requires careful thinking and planning and the decision to have sex needs to be made responsibly. Because there is no standard age when people are ready to have sex, it is important that everyone knows the dangers of unwanted pregnancies and how easily they can happen. Making love introduces a new emotional dimension into your relationship as well as bringing the risks of pregnancy. Some people may consider it unromantic to discuss contraception in advance but it is not very romantic to have an unwanted pregnancy. The better prepared you are, the more likely you will both be to find sex satisfying and pleasurable as well as safe.

Section four: THE QUESTION OF PREGNANCY

What can they tell from internal examination?

When a girl visits her doctor or family planning clinic to get contraceptives, she will be given an internal examination. The doctor will want to make sure that the visible sex organs – the vulva, vagina and cervix – have developed normally and that there is no sign of disease. The external organs are checked first for their general appearance and for things like irritation or unusual discharge. The doctor may use a finger to feel the lower end of the vagina, before inserting a speculum. This instrument is used to spread the walls of the vagina, enabling the doctor to get a clear view as far as the cervix. Mostly the findings are normal, and the doctor can see that the girl is healthy. While the speculum is in place, he or she will take a sample from the cervix for a smear test. If the girl has asked for a diaphragm, she will be measured internally for one.

After the speculum has been removed, the doctor may do what is called a bimanual examination to feel the position of the reproductive organs. This is done by putting two fingers inside the vagina and using the other hand to press on the abdomen in the region of the uterus, Fallopian tubes and ovaries.

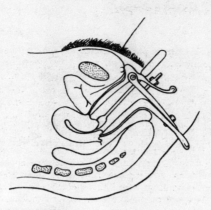

Examination using speculum

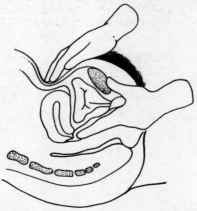

Bimanual examination

Section four: THE QUESTION OF PREGNANCY

How do I know which contraceptive works best?

Doctors and family planning clinics can help you decide which is the best contraceptive for you. The pill is the most reliable way to prevent pregnancy, so long as you remember to take it regularly. But no girl should feel that she is being forced to use the pill. It does have side-effects, like making you feel heavy or making your breasts feel sore. The condom and diaphragm (used along with a spermicide) are also effective contraceptives, but they need to be used with care each time you make love. No contraceptive works if you forget to use it.

What's a smear test and do I need one?

The smear (or Pap) test is a simple procedure for examining the cells of the cervix for any traces of disease or abnormality. All it requires is for a few cells to be taken from the surface of the cervix. This can be done during a visit to the doctor or family planning clinic and is painless. The sample taken from the cervix is sent to a laboratory where it is examined under a microscope so that any abnormality is spotted quickly.

No matter how young you are, you should have a smear test if you are already having sex. If you go to a family planning clinic, they will give you a smear test at regular intervals but you may have to ask your doctor to arrange one. It is not usually done while you are having a period.

I don't like buying condoms at the chemists. Where else can I get them?

Condoms (sheaths) are available free at family planning clinics. When girls ask for them here, they are usually given with spermicides. They are also sold in barbers and sex shops. You can buy them from slot machines in public toilets, although it is not a good idea to get them from this source: condoms perish with age, and you have no way of knowing how long they've been in the machine.

Section four: THE QUESTION OF PREGNANCY

Should a girl carry condoms?

In a relationship where you really care for each other, responsibility for contraception should be shared by both partners. Any girl who has several sex partners, or who does not use the pill or diaphragm, should probably carry some condoms with her, to make quite sure that she does not risk an unwanted pregnancy.

Don't condoms make sex less fun?

If used as a matter of routine, both partners usually become quite accustomed to the condom and don't notice its presence. Some people complain about the interruption in love-making caused by the need to put on a condom (or take it off). On the other hand, a condom reduces the fear of pregnancy, which is important if you are to enjoy sex. One way of coping is to incorporate the use of a condom into love-making: for example, the girl can help the boy put it on.

Do condoms come in different sizes?

Condoms come in different styles, textures and even colours, but they are only made in one size. The fine rubber is extremely elastic and strong. Try blowing one up like a balloon: you'll see how large it can become.

How long before sex should you put on a condom?

The time to put on a condom is as soon as the boy gets an erection, before the partners even get close to intercourse. It is better to make a habit of being prepared well in advance. This relieves the anxiety of possibly being caught out.

Section four: THE QUESTION OF PREGNANCY

How often can you use a condom?

Once only. A condom is a reasonably reliable contraceptive if it is used with a spermicide, and if it has no tears or holes in it. If a condom is damaged, it offers no protection at all.

Are condoms really safe?

Condoms are safe, but they need to be used carefully. A tear could be disastrous. Make sure no air gets trapped when the condom is rolled over the erect penis. Since a few drops of semen can leak out before ejaculation, the condom should be put on immediately the boy gets an erection. After he has 'come' (ejaculated), he should hold the condom firmly around the base of the penis and withdraw. If the condom isn't removed before the penis goes limp, there is a good chance that it will fall off. For extra safety, it is a good idea for the girl to use a spermicide as well.

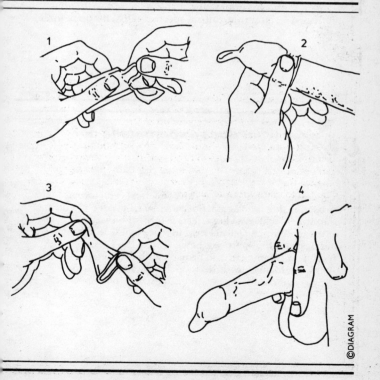

Section four: THE QUESTION OF PREGNANCY

How long do sperm live?

Once sperm have become fully developed in the boy's reproductive organs, their life-span depends on where they happen to be. Mature sperm can be stored in the seminal vesicles for several weeks before they are reabsorbed as waste by the body; sperm that are ejaculated – during masturbation, say, or a wet dream – have only a very short life. The ideal condition for the survival of sperm is a moist, warm, alkaline environment – such as is found within the uterus. Here, after intercourse, sperm can live for up to three days.

What does a spermicide do?

A spermicide kills sperm. It can come in several forms, all to be used inside the vagina. Spermicidal jelly, used inside a diaphragm, makes a very effective form of barrier contraception. The jelly is held in place by the diaphragm and destroys the sperm as they swim up the vagina. Spermicide foams can also be used with condoms. Used on their own, foams, pessaries (which dissolve inside the vagina) and creams do not give adequate protection.

I want to have sex, but I'm too frightened to go and get contraceptives. My friend says she will let me use her diaphragm. Is this safe?

If you feel that you are ready to have sex, but are not ready to accept the responsibilities, perhaps you ought to think again. If you are feeling embarrassed now, the chances are you may feel guilty later, and this is not a very good way to begin love-making. You must also accept the real risk of pregnancy, which would make you – and your boyfriend – responsible for another life as well.

It might help to talk to your boyfriend about contraception. Ask him if he will buy condoms. But it is better if you sort out your emotions and get your own contraceptives. Your friend is doing you no favours by letting you use her diaphragm. They are made in different sizes, to fit each girl, and you need to be measured for one that is right for you. And, although the diaphragm provides reliable contraception, it needs to be used with care and practice. You will be taught how to use it when you are fitted for one of your own.

Section four: THE QUESTION OF PREGNANCY

My girlfriend has a diaphragm but it looks enormous. How does she get it in?

The thick rim of the diaphragm is made of a wire coil covered with soft rubber. This makes it very flexible. When the diaphragm is inserted in the vagina, the girl just pinches the edges of the rim together and rolls it up to fit inside her.

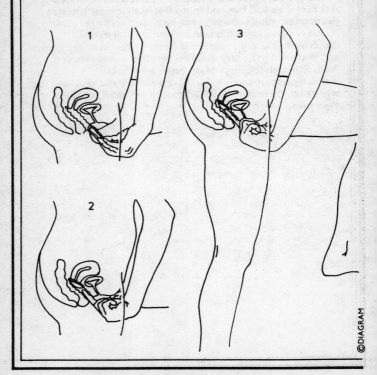

Can you have sex more than once with the diaphragm inside you, or do you have to take it out after each time?

You can leave the diaphragm in place after you've had intercourse once, but you have to use more spermicide if it has been inside you for more than three hours and you have intercourse again. After intercourse, you must leave the diaphragm in place for at least six hours, to make sure that the sperm have all been killed. Then remove the diaphragm, clean and dry it carefully and put it away.

You should, however, not leave it in for more than twenty-four hours, and it is important to follow all the instructions given when you are being fitted with one.

Section four: THE QUESTION OF PREGNANCY

How does an IUD work?

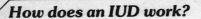

No one is sure exactly how an IUD – the intrauterine device, also known as the 'coil' – works. It is inserted into the uterus, where it can stay for as long as a few years. It seems to keep a fertilized ovum from becoming implanted in the lining of the uterus.

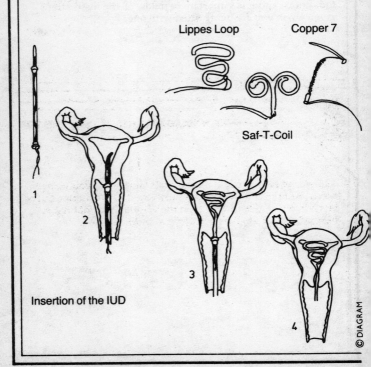

Lippes Loop

Copper 7

Saf-T-Coil

Insertion of the IUD

Is it true that IUDs can move around your body?

The only direction that an IUD can move is out through the vagina. Girls and women who have not had a baby have a uterus which is not used to having something inside it, and it may begin muscular contractions (like labour pains) to expel the IUD. This does not happen often. There is a slight chance that the IUD may cause an infection by damaging the wall of the uterus. If you are using one and start to have a lot of pain or unusual bleeding, you should see your doctor or go back to the clinic at once.

Can you use tampons if you've got an IUD?

There is no reason why you can't use tampons if you've been fitted with the coil. The IUD is positioned in the uterus, but a tampon never gets further than the vagina: it cannot travel beyond the cervix (the neck of the womb).

Section four: THE QUESTION OF PREGNANCY

Does using contraceptives stop your periods?

No contraceptive stops you from menstruating. One of the effects of the pill is to prevent the lining of the uterus from becoming thicker, so there is less bleeding every month. IUDs may cause heavier bleeding.

Why are there so many names for the pill? Are they all the same?

The contraceptive pill is made by many different drug companies, and each one has a name for its own product. But all versions of the pill are basically the same: they contain the female hormones oestrogen and progesterone (which can be combined in different amounts). They are designed to prevent ovulation, by stopping the ova (eggs) from maturing in the ovaries. It is up to your doctor to decide which is the best combination for you.

Why do you have to go to the doctor if you want to go on the pill? Why can't you just go to the chemists?

Because the pill contains powerful hormones which interrupt the normal monthly cycle, people should only take it under medical supervision. If you are healthy, do not smoke and are not overweight, the risks of being on the pill are slight. But your doctor will want to check your general health before prescribing it. And, once you go on the pill, he or she will want to check you every six months to make sure there are no side-effects.

How does the pill work? Does it kill sperm?

The pill has no effect on sperm whatsoever. It contains chemical hormones which prevent an egg from ripening and from being released from the ovary so it is impossible for conception to take place.

Section four: THE QUESTION OF PREGNANCY

Can you get addicted to the pill? Can it make you high or turn you on?

There is only one important way that the pill may affect your mind, and that is to remove the fear of pregnancy and free you to enjoy sex.

Is it possible to get pregnant on the pill?

If you take the pill as instructed, usually you will not get pregnant. If you become ill and are vomiting or have diarrhoea, then there is a good chance that your body has not been able to absorb all the hormones in each dose of the pill and you may ovulate. There are also some medicines, such as antibiotics, which may interfere with the contraceptive pill. To be safe, you must use another form of contraception for 14 days after you have recovered or have finished taking the other drug. It is always a good idea to ask your doctor about the effects of any other prescribed drug if you are on the pill.

How many times can you miss taking the pill and know that you're still safe?

It is not a good idea to miss taking the pill at all. If you accidentally forget one, take it as soon as possible. If you skip two days, then you must use another form of contraception while you finish your month's supply.

How is the mini-pill different from the pill?

The mini-pill is an oral contraceptive that contains only one hormone, progesterone. It works by changing the mucus lining the cervix, making it so thick that sperm cannot get past and enter the uterus. Since you continue to ovulate, the mini-pill acts by creating a sort of barrier and its success depends on its being taken at exactly the same time every day.

Section four: THE QUESTION OF PREGNANCY

What is the 'morning after' pill?

The 'morning after' pill is a contraceptive that is used only in emergencies. It is given by a doctor to a woman who has had intercourse, or been raped, and who is likely to become pregnant. This pill contains a large amount of hormones in a single dose and must be administered within three days, either as an injection or in a tablet form. The hormones prevent an already fertilized egg from implanting in the wall of the uterus. This massive dose has unpleasant side-effects which may last several days.

Isn't there an injection that stops you getting pregnant?

A contraceptive has been developed that can be given by injection. Depo-Provera, like the pill, contains hormones, but it is only given every three months. Doctors do not usually prescribe it, because if you develop side-effects, there is no way to withdraw the hormones from your body.

Why don't they have a pill for boys?

A pill to prevent boys producing sperm has reached trial stages. But one of the unfortunate side-effects seems to be a loss of the sex drive. At present, the condom or sheath is still the only contraceptive that can be used by boys.

I don't fancy spending years messing around with contraceptives. Can't I be sterilized and have it reversed later?

There is no short cut to effective contraception. Sterilization procedures for men and women are difficult to reverse, and usually doctors carry them out only on older people who have already had a family.

Section four: THE QUESTION OF PREGNANCY

My father has had a vasectomy. Does this mean he can't make love any more?

No, planned sterility is not the same as impotence. Vasectomy is the name given to the simple procedure for male sterilization. It involves making two small cuts in the scrotum in order to snip the duct known as the *vas deferens* on each side and tie off the cut ends (**a**). This means that, although sperm is still being produced in the testes, it can no longer make its way from there to the penis. But there is no change in sexual performance and no loss of sexual drive. Anyone who has had a vasectomy still comes in the normal way and the semen looks exactly the same as before. Vasectomy really is a very tiny operation indeed, taking only about 15 minutes, and done under a local anaesthetic so there is no pain. Many men choose to undergo it if their partners are at risk from taking the pill or to spare them the lengthier and much more serious operation for female sterilization.

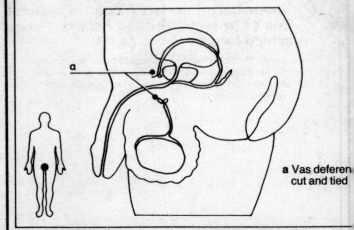

a Vas deferens cut and tied

My aunt has had her tubes tied. What does this mean?

Your aunt has had an operation to be sterilized, where the Fallopian tubes which lead from the ovaries to the uterus have been closed off permanently. This used to be done by tying and cutting the tubes. These days, they are usually sealed with clips (**a**). The operation is simple. It does not interfere with a woman's menstrual cycle – she still ovulates normally – but the egg is absorbed by the body instead of being shed during the period.

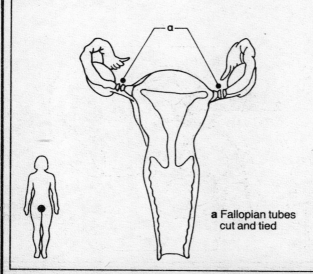

a Fallopian tubes cut and tied

Section four: THE QUESTION OF PREGNANCY

If you have sex and don't use a contraceptive, is there anything you can use afterwards to stop yourself getting pregnant?

There are several safe methods that a doctor can use if you have had intercourse and think you may become pregnant. One is the 'morning after' pill. Another is to insert an IUD, to prevent a fertilized egg from implanting in the uterus, and a third is menstrual extraction, where the lining of the uterus is removed by a suction tube inserted through the vagina. All three are emergency measures. They can only be used immediately after sex, but they cannot be regarded as a substitute for normal contraception. Nothing you can do yourself – like jumping up and down, having a hot bath or drinking a large gin – will prevent pregnancy from developing if you have conceived.

How long should you wait to find out if you're pregnant?

You should find out as soon as possible because pregnancy makes enormous demands. If an expectant mother and the developing baby in her womb are to remain healthy, she needs to take special care of herself from the very beginning, from conception. If she is very young and unmarried, she will have to decide, first of all, if she wants to continue the pregnancy, or whether she feels she must ask for a termination (abortion). The earlier this is carried out, the less risk is involved. If she decides to have her baby, she must begin to prepare for the tremendous changes brought by pregnancy – interrupting her education, for example – and must choose whether to keep her baby or offer it for adoption. If she keeps it, her life will alter dramatically. The responsibilities of motherhood are imposed by law, not just demanded by emotion. Nine months is not a long time to get ready for becoming a mother. A girl can try to ignore pregnancy, but it will not simply go away.

Section four: THE QUESTION OF PREGNANCY

I think I might be pregnant. What should I do?

The first thing is to find out as soon as possible if you really are pregnant, and that means having a pregnancy test. If you feel that you don't want to see your family doctor, you can go to a hospital, health centre or family planning clinic. The test cannot be done until 14 days after your last period was due. If the test is positive and you are under 16 or living at home, it is better to tell your parents right away; it's no use hoping they won't notice. If the test is negative, don't just breathe a sigh of relief. Make sure you use contraceptives the next time – and every time – you have intercourse.

Are home pregnancy tests reliable, or should you go to a doctor?

Do-it-yourself pregnancy tests are not reliable (partly because you are not experienced enough in laboratory techniques to carry them out correctly). You must remember that you still have to wait 14 days after the period was due before having a pregnancy test at a family planning clinic or doctor's surgery. While a positive result does mean that you are pregnant, a negative result is not an all-clear signal. You will need to wait another four or five days and then have yourself tested again to be absolutely sure.

Do you have to tell your parents if you need an abortion?

If you are under 16, you will need the written consent of your parents or legal guardian to have an abortion. No doctor will perform one without it. If you cannot face talking to your parents, you can get advice and support from a family planning clinic or from the Brook Advisory Centres.

I'm pregnant and my mother wants me to have an abortion, but I want to keep the baby. What can I do?

No one can make you have an abortion. The decision whether or not to have a baby is yours. But if you decide that you want to go ahead with the pregnancy, it is important to talk to your doctor, or you can get help from the Family Planning Association or the Brook Advisory Centres. You can also get advice from antenatal clinics.

5 Pages 144–153
Section five: GAY RELATIONSHIPS

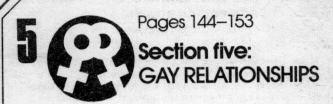

- What is homosexuality? **146**
- Why are people homosexual? **147**
- I'm attracted to an older boy/girl at school. Am I gay? **148**
- Is homosexuality on the increase? **148**
- How do gay men make love? **149**
- How do gay women make love? **149**
- Why do gays get married? **150**
- Do gays use contraceptives? **150**
- Can gays have babies? **151**
- Do gay men wish they were women? **151**
- What's the difference between a transvestite and a transsexual? **152**
- Do some people have sex with both men and women? **153**
- Are gays more promiscuous? **153**

Section five: GAY RELATIONSHIPS

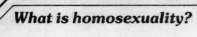

What is homosexuality?

A homosexual (from the Greek word *homos* meaning same) is a man or woman who has an emotional and sexual preference for members of his or her own sex.

Homosexuality is no longer a crime in England and Wales for consenting adults over the age of 21. It is still illegal for men under 21 to have sex with other men but it has never been considered illegal for women. Female homosexuals are often called lesbians but these days homosexuals of either sex are mostly referred to as gays.

Why are people homosexual?

The cause of homosexuality is not understood. It may be physical in some people, or psychological, or a combination of both. Discovering that you may be gay can be very difficult but there are current attempts to understand this form of sexuality and encourage greater public understanding.

Some people become homosexual because of circumstances: for example, when they are in prison for any length of time, or in a single-sex institution. They generally seek a partner of the opposite sex when they return to normal living.

Section five: GAY RELATIONSHIPS

I'm attracted to an older boy/girl at school. Am I gay?

Intense feelings for older people of the same sex are perfectly normal and common in adolescence. Don't worry: this kind of 'crush' is not an indication of your sexuality. It's just a normal – if painful – part of growing up.

Is homosexuality on the increase?

Many people think there are more gays about now that homosexuality is no longer illegal between consenting adults. And, of course, gays are more visible now that they no longer have to hide from the law. But the fact is that the proportion of gays in the community, about one in 20 people, seems to remain constant.

How do gay men make love?

Gays have the same sort of sexual relationships as heterosexuals, and as varied. How they make love is very much up to the individuals, as it is for heterosexuals. They give and get satisfaction by kissing, caressing and stimulating each other's sex organs. Some men have oral and anal intercourse, but by no means all, and it is a matter of taste and personal preference, as with all sexual relationships.

How do gay women make love?

Gay women enjoy loving and sexual relationships just like everyone else and love-making is centred around stimulation of the clitoris. How this is done is a matter of personal preference. Penis substitutes are generally not used or needed for gay women to enjoy sex.

Section five: GAY RELATIONSHIPS

Why do gays get married?

Many people (not just homosexuals) get married because of tremendous pressures to conform to what society regards as acceptable behaviour. It is not easy to be different, and, in any case, the life of a single person can be lonely. By marrying, you gain status and a level of respectability. The fact that marriage is an institution approved of and supported by law may give a married couple an added stability that is denied to unmarried couples, whether homosexual or heterosexual. Some gays may decide to marry in the hope that it will 'cure' them. However, in rare cases, marriage may bring contentment, depending on the choice of partner.

Do gays use contraceptives?

Obviously people of the same sex who make love do not need contraceptives in order to prevent pregnancy. But gay men who have anal intercourse with each other may choose to use a condom as a precaution against passing on a sexually transmitted disease.

Can gays have babies?

A gay couple cannot get pregnant together and have a baby. They may be able to adopt a child, though it is harder for gay men to do so. Gay women could get pregnant in order to have a baby, either by artificial insemination or by having sexual intercourse with a man.

Do gay men wish they were women?

No, the vast majority of gay men respond to each other sexually as men, not as substitute women. Many gay men are also good friends to women, to whom they relate quite normally as men, but without any sexual element. However, there is a small minority of men who really do feel themselves to be women trapped in male bodies. These are transsexuals – people who have the emotional make-up and identity of the opposite sex. What transsexuals are seeking is to change their sex.

Section five: GAY RELATIONSHIPS

What's the difference between a transvestite and a transsexual?

There is a big difference between transvestism and transsexuality and the two should not be confused. Transvestism (or cross-dressing) is taking physical and emotional pleasure from dressing in the clothes of the opposite sex. Most transvestites are men. But, contrary to what many people believe, transvestites are not necessarily gay. In fact, up to 75 per cent of transvestites are likely to be heterosexual (straight), leading otherwise conventional lives.

Transsexualism is altogether more complex. It is a situation where the individual feels that he or she has been born into the wrong sex. These people (and again it is more common in men) do not want to have to masquerade as a member of the opposite sex and some may want a sex-change operation. Some do indeed have the lengthy course of hormone treatment and surgery needed to bring about a sex-change.

Do some people have sex with both men and women?

Yes, they do and they are known as bisexuals (AC/DCs). They are attracted to both sexes and have sexual relationships equally with men and women. There are many others, however, who have, on occasion, been aroused by or made love to someone of their own sex as well as someone of the opposite sex but would not consider themselves bisexual.

Are gays more promiscuous?

Gays are generally no more promiscuous than heterosexuals and, once they have found a partner, live together just like any other couple. However, because of society's attitude to homosexuality, they may have difficulty finding a partner in the first place. There are, however, some gays who adopt a lifestyle that includes many and fleeting sexual encounters.

6 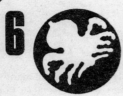 Section six: SEXUALLY TRANSMITTED DISEASES

Pages 154–173

- What are VD and STD? **156**
- What is AIDS? **157**
- What causes AIDS? **157**
- What are the symptoms of AIDS? **158**
- Can you get AIDS if you're not gay? **159**
- How can small children, and even babies, get AIDS? **159**
- What are the symptoms of syphilis? **160**
- What are the symptoms of gonorrhoea? **161**
- How do I know if I've got syphilis or gonorrhoea? **161**
- Can syphilis kill? **162**
- Can you get VD from a public lavatory? **162**
- How do you know if you've got VD or an STD? **163**
- I think I've got VD. What should I do? **164**
- What happens at a VD clinic? **165**
- If you have a vaginal discharge, does this mean you've got VD or an STD? **166**
- If you have a penis discharge, does this mean you've got VD or an STD? **166**
- What is cystitis? **167**
- How do I know if I've got cystitis? **167**
- Is cervical cancer an STD? **168**
- Do you really get cervical cancer if you have sex when you're young? **169**
- What do the initials NSU stand for? **170**
- What causes genital warts? **170**
- Someone I know says he has crabs. What does he mean? **171**
- Does kissing someone with a cold sore give you herpes? **172**
- How can you avoid getting VD? **173**

Section six: SEXUALLY TRANSMITTED DISEASES

What are VD and STD?

VD stands for venereal disease. Syphilis and gonorrhoea are two venereal diseases which are notifiable; this means they must be reported to the health authority. They can be caught only by direct sexual contact, that is, sexual intercourse, genital contact, anal contact and oral contact.

STD stands for sexually transmitted disease and includes VDs as well as other diseases which can be picked up in different ways, even if you've never had sex. Thrush, for example, is an infection caused by the imbalance of yeast or fungus which grows naturally in the vagina but can be easily cured with antibiotics. STD can apply to minor diseases and infections as well as serious ones like AIDS.

If you think you have any of the infections described here, it is important to get medical help immediately. Except for AIDS, all can be cured if detected early on and it is no good wishing or hoping they will go away. Sometimes the symptoms disappear but it does not mean the disease has gone away.

What is AIDS?

The initials AIDS stand for Acquired Immune Deficiency Sydrome, a condition where your natural defences against infection are knocked out. This means that AIDS patients are likely to get infections which the body would normally fight off. In people with lowered resistance, these can prove fatal.

AIDS victims may develop certain kinds of cancer, as well as serious infections in the lungs, skin or digestive or central nervous systems. Two diseases often found in AIDS cases (but rare in other people) are: Kaposi's sarcoma, a rare form of cancer mainly of the skin, but also affecting other parts of the body; and pneumocystis carinii pneumonia, a very serious infection of the lungs.

What causes AIDS?

AIDS is caused by a virus known to doctors as HTLV-III. When it gets into the bloodstream, it may kill off certain white blood cells which normally act to fight off germs. This leaves the body open to infections of all kinds.

But just because someone picks up the HTLV-III, it doesn't mean that he or she will automatically develop AIDS. Many thousands of people in this country are infected with the virus, but only a few hundred of these are suffering with the disease. Nobody knows why this virus makes some people ill, while others seem to remain perfectly fit.

Section six: SEXUALLY TRANSMITTED DISEASES

What are the symptoms of AIDS?

As with many illnesses, the early symptoms of AIDS are a bit vague. Taken one by one, they're the sort of thing we all get from time to time and may have nothing to do with AIDS. They include the following: **swollen glands**, especially in the neck and armpits; **profound fatigue**, which lasts for several weeks; **unexpected weight loss** – more than 10 lb in two months; **fever and sweating at night**, lasting for several weeks; **diarrhoea** which lasts for more than a week, with no obvious cause; **shortness of breath and a dry cough** lasting longer than they would if they were just from a bad cold; **marks on the skin**, pink or purple blotches which appear all over the body and look like bruises or blisters.

But, remember, each of these symptoms is quite common and may be due to some other cause. It is only when they all occur together – and last for a long time – that there may be reason for concern. Even then, only laboratory tests can show definitely whether someone has AIDS.

Can you get AIDS if you're not gay?

Yes, you can. The AIDS virus is not selective. It attacks anyone – gay or straight, boy or girl, adult or child. The groups most at risk are: homosexual and bisexual men; haemophiliacs and others who receive blood transfusions (but all donated blood is now tested before use); and drug-users who inject themselves and sexual partners of all these.

The two main ways in which the disease is passed on are: by direct sexual contact; and by getting infected blood into your bloodstream (by way of an open wound perhaps). You cannot catch the virus from toilet seats or from things like crockery or towels used by an AIDS victim.

How can small children, and even babies, get AIDS?

Assuming they haven't been assaulted by an AIDS victim, children who develop the disease do so in one of two ways. First there is the rare risk of infection from transfusions of some kind. The second route – likely to be a much bigger problem as the disease spreads – is infection from a mother who already has the AIDS virus. This deadly virus is known to be transmitted from the mother to the unborn child in the womb or at birth, or to a baby through the mother's milk.

AIDS is very rare in young children, and half the children who do contract AIDS get it in a milder form.

Section six: SEXUALLY TRANSMITTED DISEASES

What are the symptoms of syphilis?

The first sign of syphilis usually appears three to six weeks from the date of infection, but it is not always easy to detect. The first thing to look for is a small sore, a bit like a spot or cold sore, which doesn't itch or hurt. It usually appears on or near the sex organs (or it could be near the mouth), but if it develops inside the anus or vagina it will probably go unnoticed.

This first sore usually disappears after a few days or weeks, and a few more weeks will pass before the next signs appear: a copper-coloured skin rash anywhere on the body; fever, sore throat; swollen glands; and some loss of hair.

These symptoms, too, disappear eventually, and, if the condition is untreated, the next stage, a hidden one, may last for years. It gives way to the final stage of syphilis, where the disease ravages almost every organ in the body, leading to blindness, paralysis, mental collapse and death.

Fortunately, syphilis can be detected and cured in the earliest stages so, if you think you have been in contact with it, go at once for a check-up.

What are the symptoms of gonorrhoea?

Signs of gonorrhoea start to appear two to ten days after infection, but the symptoms are different for men and women. In women there may be an unusual discharge, often yellowish, from the vagina, or discharge and irritation from the anus; there may be a burning sensation on urination; and sometimes there is a slight fever, with the feelings of a chill and pains in the stomach and joints. Or women may notice no symptoms at all.

Men who catch gonorrhoea will notice: pain on urination; a yellowish discharge from the penis; and irritation and discharge from the anus.

How do I know if I've got syphilis or gonorrhoea?

These can only be caught by direct sexual contact with someone who already has them. If you think you may have been infected, even before you get any symptoms, you must get medical help immediately. If they are not treated quickly, they can become very serious. Gonorrhoea can lead to sterility in both sexes and syphilis can kill.

Section six: SEXUALLY TRANSMITTED DISEASES

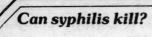

Can syphilis kill?

Untreated syphilis can kill. It is a disease which goes in stages, from minor symptoms in the early days, which can be easily treated, to terrible illness many years later.

Can you get VD from a public lavatory?

No, there is no way you can catch true venereal disease – syphilis or gonorrhoea – from indirect sources such as toilet seats or shared towels. These are diseases which you only get by direct sexual contact with someone of either sex who is already infected. Direct sexual contact includes: genital contact (when both partners' sex organs touch); anal contact (between the penis and the anus); oral contact (between the sex organs and the mouth).

How do you know if you've got VD or an STD?

The answer is you don't, or at least you can never be sure without laboratory tests. There are many different types of STD, some of which affect both sexes, some only men and some only women. No one knows where or when STDs started but the diseases have been with us for a long time. The first symptoms – such as itching, soreness, pain on urination – are often similar. Or there may be no symptoms that you can see or feel. If you notice any symptoms, or if you think you may have picked up an infection and you have had several sexual partners, go at once to your doctor or to a special clinic. Treatment and cure in the early stages is usually simple but putting off treatment can be dangerous.

Section six: SEXUALLY TRANSMITTED DISEASES

I think I've got VD. What should I do?

If you have any reason to think you have VD, or any other sexually transmitted disease, you should get help immediately. Do not panic but remember, if you delay, these conditions can be at best unpleasant and at worst a serious threat to health. The simplest thing to do is to go straight to your doctor, or to one of the clinics that specialize in diagnosing and treating sexually transmitted diseases of all kinds. They will treat you sympathetically and not make any judgments.

You can find out about these clinics from any health centre, hospital, Citizen's Advice Bureau or simply from the telephone directory; and some public lavatories have notices telling you where your nearest clinic is. It may be called a special clinic, a VD clinic or an STD clinic. If you're not sure, ask, because delay can be dangerous.

What happens at a VD clinic?

At one of these clinics you will be helped by doctors and nurses who specialize in treating STDs of all kinds. They work on a basis of strict confidentiality, both in treating you and, where necessary, in following up any of your sexual partners to try and stop the spread of disease.

On a first visit, the doctor will want to examine you thoroughly and to take a sample of blood and urine, as well as smears from the sex organs, and possibly other parts of the body, to send away for laboratory tests. On later visits, when the diagnosis is known, you will be treated and then tested again to make sure the condition is clearing up as it should.

Section six: SEXUALLY TRANSMITTED DISEASES

If you have a vaginal discharge, does this mean you've got VD or an STD?

The healthiest vagina produces a certain amount of discharge, usually clear or milky. So, discharge in itself need not be alarming unless it is dark yellow, grey or greenish in colour and smells very offensive in which case you may have a vaginal infection. But if you have a discharge together with other symptoms, such as itching in the vagina or a burning sensation when you urinate, you should seek medical advice.

If you have a penis discharge, does this mean you've got VD or an STD?

It doesn't automatically signal an infection caught by sexual contact. It could be due to a simple infection which is very common in men. But any discharge of this kind is worrying and should be investigated – and treated – at once.

What is cystitis?

Cystitis is an infection of the bladder and urethra (the tube which carries urine to the outside) in women. It is not necessarily caused by having sex, but it does often occur after love-making. It can be sexually transmitted.

Cystitis is so common that probably up to half of all women suffer it at some time in their lives; many women have repeated attacks. It is a painful condition, and there is always the risk that the infection may spread to the kidneys (particularly in young girls whose kidneys are not yet fully mature). Cystitis can be treated with antibiotics.

How do I know if I've got cystitis?

If you'd got cystitis, you could hardly settle down long enough to read this book. For this is a condition which makes you want to pee every few minutes. When you pee, it is very painful indeed – you feel a burning sensation – and there may be pus or blood in the urine. If you think you may have cystitis, drink as much fluid as you can to flush the system through and go for treatment as soon as possible.

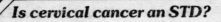

Is cervical cancer an STD?

There is a growing belief among doctors that cancer of the cervix (neck of the womb) is a disease brought about by sexual contact. This has arisen not only because it is more common in women who had frequent early sex. There is also the fact that recent research has shown that one or more viruses that are passed on during sex may be a factor in the disease. The suspects include herpes simplex virus type 2 and the virus responsible for genital warts. The evidence suggests that women are most at risk from promiscuous husbands or partners who pass on the virus infection. The risk of cervical cancer is halved if the man uses a sheath or the woman is fitted with a diaphragm. Either way, any girl or woman who is sexually active should have a smear test to detect any hint of disease at least once every five years.

Do you really get cervical cancer if you have sex when you're young?

Unfortunately, it seems that you can. Research has shown that one of the groups most at risk from cervical cancer are girls who start having sex at a very early age. The risk is greatly increased in girls who have many different sex partners. This is why many doctors now feel that (since the disease takes up to five years to develop) girls who become sexually active at 16 years or younger should have a first smear test at the latest by the age of 20. They should then be retested at frequent intervals.

Use of the sheath, or a diaphragm with spermicide, provides some protection against cervical cancer – which has been associated with a virus. And the risk is greatly reduced if neither you nor your sexual partner sleeps with anyone else and if the boy is scrupulously clean.

Section six: SEXUALLY TRANSMITTED DISEASES

What do the initials NSU stand for?

They stand for non-specific urethritis, a fairly common condition which only affects men although it can be carried by women. An infection of the tube which carries urine from the bladder to be passed out of the body, it is said to be non-specific because it isn't clear what causes it. The symptoms of NSU are the same as those for gonorrhoea – discharge from the penis and pain on urination. But, unlike VD, it is possible to pick up NSU without direct sexual contact. Women can be carriers, although they don't suffer the condition in the same way as men. So, any woman who has been in contact with an NSU-infected man should also go for treatment.

What causes genital warts?

Genital warts are fleshy growths like ordinary skin warts appearing anywhere in the genital area. They are caused by a virus, but may not begin to show for weeks or even months after you become infected. They should be treated at a special clinic, otherwise they become persistent.

Someone I know says he has crabs. What does he mean?

Crabs is another name for pubic lice, tiny parasitic insects which like to live in pubic hair especially, but which may get into the hair on other parts of the body as well. They suck blood and lay their eggs at the roots of the hair. These unwelcome guests may be picked up through direct physical contact with someone who already has them, or indirectly by using the same towels or bedding.

Pubic lice cause frantic itching which no amount of scratching or even washing will relieve. The only way to shift them is with a chemical solution available on prescription or over the counter at the chemists.

Pubic louse, greatly magnified

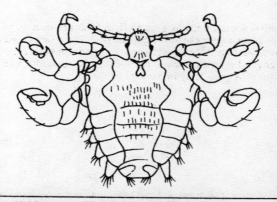

Section six: SEXUALLY TRANSMITTED DISEASES

Does kissing someone with a cold sore give you herpes?

No, it may give you cold sores but you will not get the painful and highly contagious STD known as genital herpes. The muddle arises here because the herpes cold sore virus (classified as herpes simplex virus type 1) is closely related to the type 2 virus responsible for genital herpes. But the effects of these two highly contagious viruses are different. Type 1 gives you cold sores on the mouth and you might also get 'cold sores' in the genital area if infected matter is transferred by touch. This is unpleasant but altogether different from and less serious than genital herpes. Type 2 gives you genital herpes, characterized by similar-looking sores and blisters in the genital area (which may also get transferred to the mouth, for example, during oral sex). With genital herpes you have to avoid direct physical contact, including kissing, until the sores clear up.

How can you avoid getting VD?

There is no absolutely foolproof protection against VD, except a life of celibacy (refraining from sex). But a measure of protection, often used by people who have many sexual partners (and who are, therefore, most at risk), is the sheath. In the same way, some spermicidal creams, pessaries or foams can cut down the risk and a diaphragm certainly limits the chances of a woman catching gonorrhoea.

The best protection of all is to avoid casual sex. You need have no fears in a loving relationship with a single partner you know to be free of infection.

7 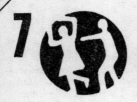 Pages 174–185
Section seven: SEX AND THE LAW

- What is the age of consent? **176**
- Is there an age of consent for boys? **176**
- Why does there have to be an age of consent? **177**
- What is paedophilia? **178**
- What's so terrible about incest? **178**
- A friend of mine is terrified of being left alone with her father because he makes advances to her. What can she do? **179**
- My uncle tries to touch me up whenever we're alone. What should I do? **180**
- The other day a man exposed himself to some of my friends in the street. Is he a rapist? **180**
- What is a voyeur? **181**
- Could a Peeping Tom turn dangerous? **181**
- What is rape? **182**
- Can you safeguard yourself against rape? **183**
- What should you do if someone tries to rape you? **184**
- Should you go to the police if you've been raped? **185**

Section seven: SEX AND THE LAW

What is the age of consent?

The age of consent is designed for the protection of young girls by the law. It is the age at which the girl can agree, legally, to have sexual intercourse: 16 years of age in England, Wales and Scotland, 17 in Northern Ireland, 18 in the Irish Republic. From the age of 14, boys can be prosecuted for having sex with under-age girls.

Is there an age of consent for boys?

No, there isn't an age of consent as such for boys, but they, too, are offered some protection by law. If an older girl or woman interferes with a boy under 16, she can be prosecuted for indecent assault. Much more common are approaches by men, which are illegal if the boy is under 21.

Why does there have to be an age of consent?

The law about sexual matters is meant for our protection, and to safeguard the young from older people who might exploit them sexually. Men having sex with under-age girls can be prosecuted for unlawful sexual intercourse (USI). Penalties vary with the age of the offender and that of the girl. The penalty for the worst sort of case, where a man has sex with a girl under 13 years of age, can be a life sentence. The girl in a case of USI is not considered to have committed a crime.

Section seven: SEX AND THE LAW

What is paedophilia?

Paedophilia comes from two Greek words which together mean the sexual love of children. This may range from petting to outright sexual abuse. In the ancient world paedophilia was widely practised, but in modern society it is seen as totally unacceptable. If caught, paedophiles, or child-molesters, face long sentences of imprisonment.

What's so terrible about incest?

Incest, which means having sexual intercourse with a close blood relative whom you cannot marry, is illegal in almost every country of the world. It leads to inbreeding which emphasizes weaknesses in a family line and stops new family units from being created.

Today, although incest rarely comes to light, it is believed still to be distressingly common, particularly between brother and sister. Many people who have been victims of incest in childhood suffer depression and other serious psychological problems in later life.

A friend of mine is terrified of being alone with her father because he makes advances to her. What can she do?

If there is a possibility of incest then the situation is very difficult. It is not easy for a young person to resist sexual approaches from a parent because the relationship between parent and child is not an equal one. The situation, however, should not be allowed to go on since it is very harmful for the child.

The dilemma your friend faces is that, if she reports this to the police, her father may be sent to prison because incest is a punishable offence. If she tells her mother, there is no guarantee what will happen. Her mother may react by being upset, angry or hurt or she may try to deny what is happening. Often in incest cases the other parent is quite unable to cope.

The best course for your friend is to tell the whole story to a sympathetic adult, someone responsible whom she can trust, like a doctor, a nurse, a minister or a teacher. Certainly, she should do something now, not let the situation get so far that it seriously undermines her health physically and psychologically.

Section seven: SEX AND THE LAW

My uncle tries to touch me up whenever we're alone. What should I do?

Many attempts at incest could be stopped with a firm 'no'. This is a furtive act, and your uncle is probably nervous and frightened of being caught out. If he tries again, tell him firmly to leave you alone and threaten to tell your parents. The threat may be enough to make him stop.

The other day a man exposed himself to some of my friends in the street. Is he a rapist?

He is what psychiatrists call an exhibitionist, someone who gets a sexual thrill from showing his penis in public and seeing the look of shock on people's faces. 'Flashers' tend to be rather timid men, unable to enjoy a normal sexual relationship. But it is not in their psychological make-up to go on to commit rape. The most effective way to deal with a flasher is to ignore him, but he should be reported to the police because indecent exposure is a crime.

What is a voyeur?

A voyeur or Peeping Tom is a person who gets sexual pleasure simply from looking at people while they are undressing, or having sex. Like flashers they are mostly timid men with severe sexual and psychological difficulties. It can be frightening to be watched and you should report them to the police since they can be charged for insulting behaviour.

Can a Peeping Tom turn dangerous?

Generally they would be much more likely to run away if challenged rather than show aggression, so they are often more of a nuisance than a danger, but in some cases they could go on to commit burglary or rape. The best defence is to make sure you cannot be seen by anyone outside your window.

Section seven: SEX AND THE LAW

What is rape?

Rape is a violent and serious crime which usually involves a man forcing a woman to have sexual intercourse against her will. Sometimes men and boys are raped also. The rapist generally threatens the victim with physical force or a weapon, but his motives are more likely to be hostility, aggression or just wanting to harm people rather than overwhelming sexual desire. Most cases of rape are premeditated and often the rapist and victim are known to each other. A rapist is dangerous and mentally sick and, if caught, can face a long prison sentence.

There are rape crisis centres which can help and give advice to rape victims. They are listed in telephone directories.

Can you safeguard yourself against rape?

Not entirely because there is no way of identifying a man as a rapist until it's too late, and girls and women of all ages are at risk. But, contrary to what you may think, most rapes do not involve complete strangers: the victim is often known to the rapist and the attack takes place at or near her home. There are various obvious precautions to be taken, like locking the house at night (and not letting in anyone you don't know) and avoiding lonely, unlit streets after dark. If you have to go home alone at night, walk briskly and purposefully – don't dawdle. More women, too, are enrolling in self-defence classes, and probably the confidence this gives them does as much to deter the would-be rapist as do the defensive skills. After all, no man is likely to attach a woman who looks fit and determined enough to hurl him over her shoulder.

Section seven: SEX AND THE LAW

What should you do if someone tries to rape you?

It's easier said than done, but the most important thing to remember is to remain as calm as you can. Don't aggravate the situation in any way. You may find that just talking to the would-be attacker quietly and making it clear that you don't want sex is enough to stop him going further. But if he does try to assault you, don't struggle unless you're fairly sure you can get away. The main thing is to get hurt as little as possible. Be passive and try to memorize details of his appearance and clothing which may help the police to track him down. If you feel you cannot talk to the police, contact a friend and tell him or her what has happened. You may need medical help to check for pregnancy, injury or a sexually transmitted disease.

Should you go to the police if you've been raped?

The decision whether to report a rape or not is almost as terrible for the victim as the crime itself. For it is well known that the police and the courts are not always as sympathetic as they might be to the victim (although this is gradually changing), and there is often the suggestion that she may have brought it on herself. It is largely for this reason that so many rapes go unreported, even though it is such a serious crime. Choosing whether to bring in the police or not is up to the victim. The investigation and subsequent court case may all be extremely unpleasant, but the victim has to remember that, if the rapist is not caught, he may do it again – and again. And, since rape is always a violent crime, someone could get killed.

GLOSSARY

Adultery: sexual intercourse between a person who is married and someone other than their husband or wife.
Anal sex: intercourse which involves putting the penis into the anus.
Aphrodisiac: a substance said to increase the sex drive.
Brothel: a place where prostitutes and their clients have sex.
Castration: removal of the testicles.
Celibacy: not having sex for a long period of time.
Cervix: the entrance to the womb.
Chastity: virginity or celibacy.
Circumcision: operation to remove the foreskin.
Clap: slang name for gonorrhoea.
Clitoris: the most sensitive part of the female body.
Coitus interruptus: withdrawal of the penis before ejaculation.
Copulation: sexual intercourse.
Crabs: pubic lice.
Cunnilingus: stimulation with the mouth of female genitals.
Curse: slang name for periods (menstruation).
Dutch cap (diaphragm): one of the barrier methods of birth control.
Embryo: an unborn child in the first two months of pregnancy.
Endometrium: the lining of the womb.
Epididymis: organ at the top of the testicle where sperm are stored.
Erotic: sexually stimulating.
Fallopian tubes: tubes leading from the ovaries to the uterus.
Family planning: birth control.
Fellatio: stimulation of the penis with the mouth.
Fertilization: a sperm meeting a ripe egg cell – the moment a baby is conceived.
Flasher: a person who gets pleasure by showing his genitals in public.
Foetus: an unborn child after the second month of pregnancy.
Foreplay: stimulation before intercourse to prepare the body and give pleasure.
French letter: slang name for sheath (condom).
Genitals: the external sex organs.
Gonads: the primary sex organs; ovaries in women and testicles in men.
Gonorrhoea: a sexually transmitted disease.
Gynaecology: the branch of medicine concerned with the female reproductive system.
Hermaphrodite: someone with both male and female sexual features.
Herpes: genital herpes (type 2) is a sexually transmitted disease.
Herpes simplex: (type 1) is a cold sore.

Hysterectomy: removal of a woman's uterus.
Implantation: when a fertilized egg becomes fixed in the wall of the uterus.
Impotence: a man's inability to have an erection or orgasm.
Incest: illegal sexual intercourse between close relatives, eg. brother and sister, father and daughter.
IUD: intrauterine contraceptive device.
Labia: the folds of skin outside the vagina.
Libido: the urge to be sexually active.
Male chauvinist pig: a man who has sexist views about the role of women.
Masochist: someone who gets pleasure from having pain inflicted on him or her.
Missionary position: the most common position for sexual intercourse with the couple lying face to face, with the man on top.
Molest: to make unwanted sexual advances.
NSU: Non-specific urethritis, a sexually transmitted disease affecting men only.
Nocturnal emission: a wet dream.
Nymphomaniac: a woman with excessive sexual desires.
Oral sex: stimulation of the sex organs with the mouth.
Ovaries: two small organs at either side of the uterus where eggs are produced.
Ovum (plural ova): Latin for egg. An ovum is released from the ovary once a month (ovulation).
Paedophile: an adult who is sexually attracted to children.
Perversion: atypical sexual activity.
Petting: a general term for kissing and touching but does not include intercourse.
Phallus: a non-medical term for the penis.
Platonic friendship: one that does not involve sex.
Pornography (porn): pictures, writings, films intended to be sexually stimulating.
Pox: slang name for syphilis.
Premature ejaculation: coming too soon.
Premenstrual tension (PMT): pain and discomfort felt by some women just before a period.
Progesterone: hormone which stimulates lining of the uterus to receive a fertilized egg. One of the ingredients of the contraceptive pill.
Promiscuity: sexual intercourse with several different acquaintances over a short period of time.
Prostate gland: one of the male sex organs which lies beneath the bladder and produces fluid which mixes with semen.
Prostitute: someone who has sexual intercourse in return for money.
Pubic lice: a sexually transmitted disease caused by a bloodsucker, the crab louse which lives in pubic hair.
Rape: a serious crime in which a person is forced to have sexual intercourse against their will.

Reproduction: production of offspring.
Rhythm method: a method of contraception based on only having sexual intercourse when the woman is least likely to conceive.
Sadist: someone who gets pleasure from inflicting pain on others.
Scabies (itch): a skin disease caused by a mite which burrows under the skin, usually between fingers, around the waist, in the armpits or groin. Can be caught through sexual contact.
Seminal vesicles: where sperm mixed with fluid from the prostate gland is stored.
Sexist: someone who thinks that people should behave in a particular way because of their sex.
Sexual harassment: making unwanted sexual advances towards someone.
Sixty-nine: simultaneous oral sex, the bodies making the shape of 69.
Snogging: similar to petting.
Sodomy: anal intercourse.
Solicit: to approach people in public offering sex in return for payment. It is a legal offence.
Spermatozoon (sperm): the male sex cells.
Sterility: the inability to have children.
Syphilis: a serious sexually transmitted disease. Now fairly rare.
Testicle (testis): the male sex organ where sperm are produced.
Thrush (candidosis): a common sexually transmitted disease but one which can develop without sexual contact. It usually only affects females and can be easily cleared up with antibiotics.
Transsexual: someone who wants to change sex.
Transvestite: someone who wears clothing of the opposite sex.
Trichomoniasis (trich or TV): a sexually transmitted disease. In women it causes infection of the vagina but can cause bladder infection in both sexes.
Umbilicus: the navel.
Urethra: the tube which carries urine from the bladder to the outside of the body.
Ureter: the tubes which carry urine from the kidney to the bladder.
Uterus (womb): the female sex organ where a baby grows.
Vagina: the tube leading from the uterus to the outside of the female body.
Vaginissmus: severe contraction of the walls of the vagina, making intercourse difficult or impossible.
Vas deferens (seminal duct): tubes which carry sperm from the epididymis (where they are stored) to the prostate gland (where they mix with seminal fluid).
Virgin: someone who has never had sexual intercourse.
Voyeur (Peeping Tom): someone who gets pleasure from watching other people undressing or having sex.
Vulva: the external female genitals.
Whore: a prostitute.
Withdrawal method: method of contraception when the man withdraws his penis from the vagina before ejaculation.

INDEX

A
Abortion, 141, 143
AC/DC, 153
Adolescence, 37
Age of consent, 16, 176, 177
AIDS, 156–159
  and children, 159
  and heterosexuals, 159
  symptoms, 158
  what causes it?, 157, 159
  what is it?, 157
Alcohol and sex, 102
Anal sex, 112

B
Bimanual examination, 118–119
Bisexuality (AC/DC), 153
Boredom with sex, 87
Bras, 61
Breast size, 59, 60
Breast cancer, 62, 63
Breast examination, 62
Breastfeeding, 61
Breasts, men's, 63, 77

C
Cancer,
  breast, 62, 63
  cervical, 168, 169
  smear test, 120
Circumcision, 102, 186
Clinics, VD, 164, 165
Clitoris, 56–57
Cold sores, 172
Coming (see Orgasm)
Condoms,
  buying, 17, 121
  effects on pleasure, 122
  how to put on, 124–125
  safety of, 124–125
  should girls carry?, 122
  size of, 123
  used only once, 124
  when to put on, 123
Contraception,
  after sex, 136, 140
  choosing best method, 121
  condoms, 17, 121, 122, 123, 124–125
  Depo-Provera, 136
  diaphragm, 127, 128, 129
  and gay sex, 150
  injections, 136
  IUD, 130, 131, 140
  mini-pill, 135
  'morning after' pill, 136, 140
  and periods, 114–115, 116, 132
  the pill, 132, 133, 134, 135
  pill for men, 137
  safe period, 114–115
  sex without, 113
  spermicide, 126
  sterilization, 137, 138, 139
  and tampons, 114
  teaching about, 117
  vasectomy, 138
Crabs, 171
Cystitis, 167

D
Deodorants, vaginal, 59
Depo-Provera, 136
Diaphragm, 127, 128, 129

Disabled people and sex, 30
Discharge from genitals, 166
Disease, sexually transmitted, (see STD)

E
Eggs, 43, 44
Ejaculation, 71, 72–73
Erection, 72–73, 74, 75, 84, 94
Erogenous zones, 83
Exhibitionists, 180

F
Family planning clinics, 118, 121, 142
Fertility, 43, 55
First time, 86, 109
Flashers, 180
French kissing, 24
Frigidity, 20, 21

G
Genital warts, 170
Gonorrhoea, 161

H
Herpes, 172
Hips, 40–41
Homosexuality, 144–153
 am I gay?, 148
 bisexuals (AC/DCs), 153
 gays and babies, 151
 increase in, 148
 and marriage, 150
 and promiscuity, 153
 reasons for, 147
 gay sex acts, 149
 transsexuals, 151, 152
 what is it?, 146
HTLV-III, 157

I
Illness, 99
Impotence, 95, 96
Incest, 178, 179, 180
Indecent exposure, 180
Infertility, 55
Internal examination, 118–119
IUD (Intrauterine device), 130, 131, 132, 140

K
Kissing and herpes, 172

L
Law and sex, 174–185
Love, being in, 25, 26
Love bites, 105

M
Masturbation, 29, 80, 81, 82
Mini-pill, 135
Missionary position, 104

N
Nipples, 61, 62, 84
NSU (Non-specific urethritis), 170
Nymphomania, 23

O
Older boyfriends, 29
Oral sex, 92, 98, 112
Orgasm, 88–92
 coming too soon, 93
 frequency of, 91, 93

knowing if you've had one, 88
not coming, 89, 90
and pregnancy, 110–111
Ovulation, 43, 44

P

Paedophilia, 178
Pain, during sex, 86
Parents
and abortion, 143
and daughters, 28
embarrassment about sex, 27
and grandparents' remarriage, 31
and incest, 179
knowing if you have sex, 104
and older boyfriends, 29
sex lives of, 30
Peeping Toms, 181
Penis discharge, 166
Penis size, 64–65
Periods, 45–50
and contraceptives, 132
irregular, 46–47, 54, 116
missed, and pregnancy, 54
premenstrual tension, 49
and pregnancy, 113
sex during, 98
Perversion, 33
Petting, and testicles, 85
Pill the,
effectiveness, 134, 135
how it works, 133
how to get it, 133
for men, 137
the 'morning after' pill, 136, 140
problems, 134
types, 132
PMT (Premenstrual tension), 49
Pregnancy, 106–143
and anal sex, 112
and the first time, 109
and oral sex, 112
and orgasm, 110–111
and periods, 113
and sex standing up, 109
sex without contraceptives, 113
tests, 142
and virginity, 108
waiting to find out, 141
what to do, 142
(see also Contraception)
Premenstrual tension (PMT), 49
Promiscuity, 19, 20,
and gays, 153
Prostitutes, 32
Puberty, 36, 37
Pubic hair, 37, 38–39
Pubic lice, 171

R

Rape,
avoiding, 183, 184
and the police, 185
what is it?, 182

S

Safe period, 114–115
Semen, and urine, 77
(see also Sperm)
Sex act,
duration, 87
first time, 86, 109
frequency, 100
gay men and women, 149

good lovers, 100–103
and pain, 86
right and wrong sex, 31, 33
Sexually transmitted disease
(see STD)
Sheath (see Condom)
Sixty-nine, 98
Smear test, 120
Speculum, 118–119
Sperm, 69, 70, 71, 126
and the pill, 133
semen and urine, 77
Spermicide, 126
STD, (Sexually Transmitted
Disease) 99, 154–173
AIDS, 156, 157, 158, 159
avoiding, 173
crabs, 171
genital warts, 170
gonorrhoea, 161
knowing if you've got it,
163
NSU, 170
and public lavatories, 162
syphilis, 160, 161, 162
VD clinics, 164, 165
what to do, 164
Sterility, 96
and gonorrhoea, 161
Sterilization, 137, 138
139
Syphilis, 160, 161, 162

T

Tampons, 50–53
and contraception, 114
and IUDs, 131
Testicles,
aching after petting, 85
different sizes, 66–67
importance of, 66–67

and sperm, 69
undescended, 68
Transsexuals, 151, 152
Transvestites, 152
Tubes, tying, 139

V

Vaginal discharge, 166
Vasectomy, 138
Venereal Disease (VD – see
gonorrhoea, syphilis
and STD)
Voice, breaking, 40–41
Voyeurs, 181

W

Warts, genital, 170
Wet dreams, 58, 75, 76
Wetness, in girls, 58
Womb, 42, 44